CMT Exam Guide

A Walk Through the Blue Print

The Association for Healthcare Documentation Integrity

Rebecca McSwain, PhD, CMT
Lea Sims, CMT, AHDI-F
Kristin Wall, CMT, AHDI-F

ahdi

Publisher: Association for Healthcare Documentation Integrity
Authors: Rebecca McSwain, PhD, CMT; Lea M. Sims, CMT, AHDI-F; Kristin Wall, CMT, AHDI-F
Managing Editor: Lea M. Sims, CMT, AHDI-F
Copyeditors: Kristin Wall, CMT, AHDI-F; Rebecca McSwain, PhD, CMT
Professional Programs Manager: Kelly Kappmeier
Interior Design: Lea M. Sims, CMT, AHDI-F
Cover Design: Network Media Partners, Inc.
Printer: CADMUS, Port City Press – A Cenveo Company

AHDI
4230 Kiernan Avenue, Suite 130
Modesto, CA 95356
800-982-2182
www.ahdionline.org

CADMUS, Port City Press
1323 Greenwood Rd.
Baltimore, MD 21208

DISCLAIMER

Care has been taken to confirm the accuracy of the information present and to describe generally accepted practices and represent common practical scenarios. However, the authors, editors, and publisher are not responsible for errors or omissions or for any consequences from application of the information in this book and make no warranty, expressed or implied, with respect to the currency, completeness, or accuracy of the contents of the publication. Application of this information in a particular situation remains the professional responsibility of the practitioner.

ISBN 978-0-935229-62-2

Printed in the United States of America

To purchase additional copies of this book, call our member services department at (800) 982-2182 or purchase this text online at www.ahdionline.org.

Look for AHDI on Facebook, Twitter, and Linked In under *Association for Healthcare Documentation Integrity*. Visit our blog at www.ahdilounge.blogspot.com.

"You cannot teach a man anything;
you can only help him find it within himself."

– Galileo Galilei
(1564-1642)

Table of Contents

Acknowledgements

On behalf of AHDI, I would like to extend our gratitude to the following association leaders and experts who assisted in the preparation of this workbook through blue print item-writing. As always, we are appreciative of the passion these individuals have for preparing our next generation workforce for professional credentialing:

Kim Buchanan, CMT, AHDI-F
Lisa Day Johnson, CMT, AHDI-F
Judith Lichtenberger, RHIT, CMT, AHDI-F
Amy Potter, CMT
Glenda Ripley, CMT
Beth Sutherland, CMT, MA

In addition, we would like to acknowledge the hard work and contributions of our Professional Programs staff, outstanding team players who made sure we met our deadlines for this manuscript:

- *Laura Bryan, MT (ASCP), CMT, AHDI-F* for her oversight and guidance in making sure the content complied with our exam blue print and represented the intent and scope of our objectives for CMT candidates.

- *Kelly Kappmeier* for applying her project management training and organizational skills to execute this text on a fast-track schedule.

- *Tina Wilson* for much-needed support and coordination as well as excellent oversight of other departmental priorities while our professional staff focused on this manuscript.

Thank you to the 2010 House of Delegates, who acknowledged the important goal of legitimizing transcription/editing as a risk management and regulatory compliance profession by passing a resolution in August 2010 that called for the mandatory credentialing of all professionals who have access to protected health information through the documentation process.

Finally, to the authors of this text—*Rebecca McSwain, PhD, CMT,* and *Kristin Wall, CMT, AHDI-F*—thank you for your focus, hard work, and expertise in developing this text. No book can adequately cover the breadth of knowledge and experience needed for a high-stakes credentialing exam, but you have created a great framework here to assist candidates in preparation, one that truly enables them to have a strategic approach to studying against the exam blue print.

Lea M. Sims, CMT, AHDI-F
Director of Professional Programs, AHDI

How to Use This Book

This text is designed to be used as a supplemental study guide in preparation for the AHDI Certified Medical Transcriptionist (CMT) exam. Students and practitioners who seek access to the CMT exam need to begin that process of preparation with a strong orientation to the exam blue print.

This book provides potential exam candidates with a "walk through the blue print," the goal of which is to make sure that the CMT candidate has a clear understanding of the industry's expectations of competency for a Level 2 candidate and the content domains against which a candidate will be evaluated on the exam. It is, by design, an orientation specifically to the cognitive assessment (multiple-choice) objectives housed on the blue print.[1]

Each chapter contains a *Chapter Overview* to orient the reader to exam objectives and competencies being addressed in the chapter as well as a bulleted list of what skills related to those objectives are critical to the execution of the MT/editor skill set at Level 2. Beyond that, each chapter offers the following organizational approach to intentional, focused study for each CMT objective covered in the chapter:

- *Statement of Objective* from the CMT Blue Print
- *Rationale* that explains the importance of that exam objective and why its inclusion on the exam blue print is important for demonstrating Level 2 competency as a CMT
- *Recommendations for Focused Study,* with a list of recommended texts and corresponding chapters and sections to aid in directed study against the blue print objective
- *Sample Questions* that demonstrate the scope and format of potential exam questions and give the candidate a feel for the type of questions that may be asked under that blue print objective

Once a candidate has worked his/her way through this guide, the text will offer a *Practice Test,* a 78-question test designed to simulate the weight and balance of cognitive assessment (multiple-choice) items found on the CMT exam and allow the candidate to diagnose areas of weakness and assess needs for further study.

Housed in the appendices of this text is a full copy of the CMT blue print (*See: Appendix B: CMT Blue Print Check List*) formatted to allow candidates to check off each blue print objective when it has been studied and mastered. The appendices also contain other valuable resources related to AHDI credentialing exams and assessment aids and products. If you have any questions or need further assistance related to this text, please feel free to forward your inquiries to credentialing@ahdionline.org.

---

[1] The audio objectives on the CMT Blue Print are **not** addressed here but will be addressed in the audio volume of this text to be published/released at a later date.

Foreword

Three letters. Just three. What can three letters do? Quite simply, they tell others that you have passed a test. But those three simple letters after your name do more than add to your signature line. They raise your personal bar and lift an entire industry—one person at a time.

What would those three letters mean to you? Many people seek certification because of the potential for higher pay, but those who have achieved it talk about more than just their paycheck. They often speak of the pride of accomplishment or the triumph of conquering their fear of tests. Some CMTs delight in outwardly validating what they inwardly knew about themselves, while others take satisfaction in their new-found self-esteem. Some transcriptionists speak of the credibility that comes with those three little letters that follow their name. And yet others value the increased opportunities and open doors afforded by the credential. Attaining these three little letters will take on a unique and personal meaning for you, too.

No doubt, the tangible and intangible benefits of certification are both personally rewarding and professionally valuable, but one must not overlook the benefit of a credentialing program to the workforce as a whole. For all that these letters can do for the individual, a widely embraced certification program does even more for the profession. The meticulous process of developing a certification program identifies, defines, and catalogues the tangible knowledge and skills required to perform the job. The certification blue print reveals the complexity of what might appear to be mundane work by outlining the in-depth language skills, extensive medical terminology, and the range of technical knowledge required to practice successfully in this field.

For a widely misunderstood and practically invisible job such as medical transcription, defining the fund of knowledge is perhaps the most important aspect of a credentialing program. As transcriptionists, we have been plagued by the over-simplification of our skills and the constant harassment of speech recognition technology that has been touted to cheaply and irreverently replace us. Our certification program draws attention to the complexity and nuanced skills that come from a blending of talent, education, experience, and commitment to continuing education. Within the healthcare industry, certification is a widely recognized method of verifying competency, and the letters RMT and CMT succinctly communicate to others that we possess identifiable skills and explicit knowledge that extend far beyond our keyboarding ability.

A successful certification program is like a tide that raises all ships. By participating in the certification program, you help elevate the entire profession. Reaching a critical mass of certified transcriptionists will allow the marketplace to finally realize the true benefits of a credentialed workforce. While certification programs in general are intended to promote public safety by ensuring a qualified workforce, the achievement of industry-mandated certification of the transcription workforce will have even more impact. A well-designed certification program that is widely accepted by practitioners and employers extracts accountability from educators, employers, and individual practitioners alike. It also creates barriers that protect professional practitioners from an influx of unqualified workers that encourages wage compression.

Certification also creates opportunity. It communicates to those outside our field our fundamental skills and how those skills can translate to emerging roles in healthcare documentation. To an industry that has become acutely focused on the privacy and security of patient information, a credential that assesses knowledge of federal statutes such as HIPAA can serve as a key to unlocking jobs in the field of health information management.

To accomplish its goals, a certification program should give practical guidance for hiring and staffing decisions. The 2011 release of the RMT and CMT exams corresponds to the Association for Healthcare Documentation Integrity's Level 2 job descriptions for medical transcriptionists. The RMT exam assesses fundamental knowledge of grammar, medical terminology, technology, and medicolegal guidelines. The CMT exam is designed to test knowledge that comes from practical experience, indicating mastery of the craft beyond the textbook. The CMT implies a level of experience that enables critical thinking, problem solving, and risk management. As such, the two tests can be used as tools for planning your career trajectory.

To add more value to the RMT and CMT credentials, AHDI continues to evolve its certification program to reflect changes in the industry. The HITECH Act and the electronic health record are washing over the healthcare industry like a tsunami, dramatically changing the way providers document the delivery of care. In response to this changing landscape, the 2011 release of the CMT exam includes a new section on health information technology that assesses knowledge of the electronic health record, speech recognition technology, and medical nomenclatures. This addition to the certification test emphasizes the need for practitioners to prepare for the technological changes that are impacting medical transcription and demonstrates to the healthcare industry at large that our workforce is primed and ready to participate in the new healthcare documentation paradigm.

As you work through this blue print and prepare for the certification exam, take pride in your depth of knowledge. Be encouraged by what you already know and be excited about what you learn in the process. You will discover that they are not just three little letters; they are powerful letters. Find out what these letters mean to you and let these three letters carry you on a wave of professional success!

Best wishes to you in all your endeavors.

Laura Bryan, MT (ASCP), CMT, AHDI-F
2011 Chair, AHDI Credentialing Development Team

Section 1

Clinical Medicine

"Becoming a CMT has provided the opportunity for me to pursue my true passion—teaching! Having the CMT credential was mandatory. Being credentialed is the way that I validate what I have learned—through formal education, through self-study, and on the job over the last 10+ years. Earning and maintaining my credential provides the way for me to confidently say, yes, I have a verifiable skill set, I know what I'm doing, and I do it well." – Susan Whatley, CMT, AHDI-F

Medical Terminology
Beyond the Basics

Certified Medical Transcriptionist

Chapter 1

EXAM BLUE PRINT

"In every kind of communication...from a prescription for a controlled substance to instructions for assembling a bicycle...the transmission of meaning demands consistency and precision in the use of language."

– John H. Dirckx, MD, "Foreword," ***The Book of Style for Medical Transcription, Third Edition***

Chapter Overview

At the entry level, a medical transcriptionist comes into the documentation process with a solid knowledge of medical terminology, understanding the etymology of medical words, the rules of formation for medical terms, and possessing a basic lexicon for the language of medicine. After two or more years of acute-care experience, the transcriptionist has begun to acquire a more nuanced and broader understanding of usages and meanings of medical terms and to appreciate the range of variation in usage among individual healthcare providers. At this level, a medical transcriptionist is prepared to avoid or correct errors and to enhance patient safety and the quality of medical care regardless of the mode of creation of the medical document. Further, the experienced transcriptionist is able to achieve document integrity and clarity without compromising the unique voice of the document originator or the uniqueness of the individual patient health story.

The body of knowledge in medical terminology expected of acute-care medical transcriptionists therefore includes an understanding of:

- Critical differences in terms misused or confused with others in multiple specialties and acute-care contexts.
- The correct expansion of abbreviations used in a range of specialties and acute-care contexts.

There are **2 objectives**[1] on the CMT blue print that address concepts related to these domains and against which a CMT exam candidate will be evaluated. In this chapter, we will walk through each objective listed under *CMT Blue Print Section 1: Clinical Medicine* that relates to these terminology domains.

Objective 1.1

Objective 1.1: *Given a sentence, identify the correct use of a commonly confused medical term.*

Rationale

Though medical communication relies upon clarity and lack of ambiguity, the acute-care transcriptionist is alert to the fact that there is a group of terms within any specialty area that can be misused, confused with other terms, or misunderstood in the process of transcription, whether traditional or speech-recognized. While respecting the fact that the healthcare provider has ultimate legal responsibility for the accuracy of the record, the transcriptionist is able to assist the document originator to maintain both accuracy and intelligibility in the use of medical terminology.

Recommendations for Focused Study

1. *The Book of Style for Medical Transcription, Third Edition*; Appendix C: Usage Glossary

---

[1] Objective 1.2 on the CMT blue print is an audio objective that also relates to medical terminology beyond the basics. Look for blue print guidance on audio objectives in upcoming AHDI exam prep products.

2. *The Language of Medicine, 9th Edition,* Davi-Ellen Chabner (Elsevier)

Sample Questions

Each question below represents the kind of format and content, per the exam blue print, that a CMT candidate can expect to find on the CMT exam. *Note: These are sample questions only. They are questions that do not currently appear on the CMT exam. Though some may represent items retired from previous exam forms, not all items have been psychometrically analyzed, and AHDI cautions candidates against the presumption that these items alone may be diagnostic or indicative of candidate performance.* **(Answer key at end of chapter.)**

1. Which sentence is correctly transcribed?

   A. Plain x-ray of the lower extremity showed a fracture of the malleus.
   B. Plane x-ray of the lower extremity showed a fracture of the malleus.
   C. Plain x-ray of the lower extremity showed a fracture of the malleolus.
   D. Plane x-ray of the lower extremity showed a fracture of the malleolus.

2. Which sentence is correctly transcribed?

   A. Recanalization of both vas deferens had occurred.
   B. Recanalization of both vasa deferentia had occurred.
   C. Rechannelization of both vas deferens had occurred
   D. Rechannelization of both vas deferentia had occurred.

3. Choose the correctly transcribed sentence.

   A. Imaging showed an area of plague with vessel remottling.
   B. Imaging showed an area of plaque with vessel remottling.
   C. Imaging showed an area of plaque with vessel remodeling.
   D. Imagining showed an area of plaque with vessel remodeling.

4. Which phrase correctly uses the medical term?

   A. actinic cell carcinoma
   B. acinic ketosis
   C. acinic keratosis

D. actinic keratosis

5. Which is correctly transcribed?

A. The pathology report showed a high mitotic rate.
B. Pupillometry showed that mitosis occurred.
C. The process of miosis produces sperm cells.
D. Mitosis may be a side effect of opioid use.

Objective 1.11

Objective 1.11: *Given an abbreviation, identify the correct term, or given a term, identify the correct abbreviation.*

Rationale

Not only are there abbreviations widely used in medical practice in general, but also each clinical area has its own set of more or less commonly understood abbreviations. Moving into more focused acute-care practice, the transcriptionist must acquire an enlarged abbreviations vocabulary pertaining to a variety of specialties.

Recommendations for Focused Study

1. *The Book of Style for Medical Transcription, Third Edition*; Section 4
2. *Using Medical Terminology: A Practical Approach,* J.L. Nath (Lippincott Williams & Wilkins); "Common Abbreviations" section in each specialty chapter.
3. *The Language of Medicine, 9th Edition*, Davi-Ellen Chabner (Elsevier).

Sample Questions

Each question below represents the kind of format and content, per the exam blue print, that a CMT candidate can expect to find on the CMT exam. *Note: These are sample questions only. They are questions that do not currently appear on the CMT exam. Though some may represent items retired from previous exam forms, not all items have been psychometrically analyzed, and AHDI cautions candidates against the presumption that these items alone may be diagnostic or indicative of candidate performance.* (**Answer key at end of chapter.**)

6. In neurology, what is an abbreviation for a test that measures stimulated electrical signals?

A. BNP
B. PGF
C. BSER
D. BAEP

7. What is the correct meaning of TIMI?

A. thrombosis in myocardial infarction
B. thrombin inhibition in myocardial infarction
C. thrombolysis in myocardial infarction
D. transmural inferior myocardial infarction

8. In the context of a sleep study, what does the acronym REM stand for?

A. regular eye motion
B. random eye movement
C. rapid eye movement
D. repeating eye motion

9. For which medical specialty would the abbreviation SLR be likely to be found in the physical exam?

A. neurology
B. infectious disease
C. obstetrics
D. psychiatry

10. In neonatology, what does CRL mean?

A. chest, ribs, lungs
B. crown-rump length
C. cranium-rump length
D. critical restriction limits

Sample Questions Answer Key

1. C
2. B
3. C
4. D
5. A
6. D
7. C
8. C
9. A
10. B

Certified Medical Transcriptionist

Chapter 2

EXAM BLUE PRINT

Understanding Clinical Diagnostics

"Flagging inconsistencies and discrepancies in the health record is the guardian role of the MT, and providers rely on the keen eyes, ears, and interpretive mind of the MT to ensure that health data is captured and recorded accurately, that inconsistencies are addressed, and that the amended record is authenticated by the provider."

– **"The Case for a Credentialed Workforce"**

Chapter Overview

The process of medical decision-making often begins with an analysis of signs, symptoms, patient history, and a physical examination, and then turns to the acquisition of objective diagnostic data from laboratory and imaging studies. At the beginning of a medical transcription career, the practitioner is expected to have a working knowledge of the basic vocabulary of clinical diagnostics: terms that relate to laboratory tests, procedures, and results, and terms relating to imaging studies, procedures, and results. After two years or more of experience in an acute-care setting, the transcriptionist will have built on this basic fund of information to broaden his or her understanding to include a considerable variety of laboratory tests and imaging studies. The Level 2 transcriptionist also has acquired an understanding and appreciation of the relationships among diagnostic tests and diagnoses, will have an immediate command of what laboratory and imaging study results mean, and will be able to employ the correct expression of those results.

The body of knowledge in clinical diagnostics for acute-care medical transcriptionists therefore includes an understanding of:

- Normal values for a range of laboratory tests.
- Processes, technologies, and patient positions for a variety of imaging studies used in multiple specialties.
- The kinds of contrast media used in imaging studies in various specialty applications.
- The relationship between particular imaging studies and specific diseases and diagnoses.
- Definitions and correct expression of imaging study values.
- What is being measured on any given laboratory or other diagnostic test.
- The relationship between a test or set of values and specific diseases and diagnoses for any given laboratory test or set of values.

There are **7 objectives**[1] on the CMT blue print that address concepts related to these domains and against which a CMT exam candidate will be evaluated. In this chapter, we will walk through each objective listed under *CMT Blue Print Section 1: Clinical Medicine* that relates to these clinical diagnostic domains.

Objectives 1.3, 1.18, and 1.19

Objective 1.3: *Given a laboratory result, identify if the value is low, high, or normal.*

Objective 1.18: *Given a diagnostic test including laboratory studies, identify what is being measured.*

Objective 1.19: *Given laboratory test results or values, identify the associated disease or diagnosis, or given a disease or diagnosis, identify the associated laboratory test results or values.*

[1] Objectives 1.4, 1.9, and 1.20 on the CMT blue print are audio objectives that also relate to Understanding Clinical Diagnostics. Look for blue print guidance on audio objectives in upcoming AHDI exam prep products.

Rationale

Considering the importance of laboratory results in the diagnostic process and in decision-making about treatment, and given the assumed objective precision of laboratory values, accuracy is essential when these data are introduced into a patient's healthcare record. With the advent of the electronic record, any unchecked error in laboratory data can be introduced into a document immediately usable by anyone in the wider healthcare system involved in that patient's care, thus perpetuating and reinforcing that error. In our role as collaborator in the guardianship of documentation accuracy, acute-care transcriptionists/editors must know the range of normal values for a wide variety of laboratory results. Additionally, in the interest of accuracy and document integrity, the experienced practitioner will have a fundamental understanding of the underlying meaning of laboratory test procedures and results, and will be able to relate specific laboratory tests to specific diseases, conditions, and diagnoses.

Recommendations for Focused Study

1. *The Book of Style for Medical Transcription, Third Edition*; Chapters 14 – 24.
2. *Laboratory Tests and Diagnostic Procedures in Medicine*, J. H. Dirckx (Health Professions Institute)
3. *The CMT Review Guide* (Stedman's); Appendix 1
4. *Human Diseases, Third Edition*, J. H. Dirckx (Health Professions Institute)

Sample Questions

Each question below represents the kind of format and content, per the exam blue print, that a CMT candidate can expect to find on the CMT exam. *Note: These are sample questions only. They are questions that do not currently appear on the CMT exam. Though some may represent items retired from previous exam forms, not all items have been psychometrically analyzed, and AHDI cautions candidates against the presumption that these items alone may be diagnostic or indicative of candidate performance.* **(Answer key at end of chapter.)**

1. What is the significance of a PT value of 25 seconds?

   A. Prothrombin time is increased.
   B. Prothrombin time is normal.

C. Partial thromboplastin time is increased.
D. Partial thromboplastin time is normal.

2. On tonometry testing, what is the range of normal values for IOP?

A. 10-21 mmHg
B. 100-150 mmHg
C. 500-700 mmHg
D. 1000-1500 mmHg

3. What is the purpose of a VDRL test?

A. To evaluate for any STD
B. Evaluation for HIV
C. To evaluate for syphilis
D. Evaluation for gonorrhea

4. What does the value of GFR indicate?

A. Progression of a radioisotope through the kidneys
B. Rate at which blood is filtered at the glomeruli
C. The amount of protein in urine
D. The stage of kidney disease

5. On echocardiogram, what is evaluated using a mean pressure gradient measurement?

A. ventricular hypertrophy
B. atrial hypertrophy
C. coronary artery narrowing
D. aortic valve stenosis

6. What condition is suspected in a patient with a decreased albumin and an increased ALT?

A. ketoacidosis
B. primary liver disease
C. chronic obstructive pulmonary disease
D. sclerosing cholangitis

Objectives 1.5, 1.6, 1.7, and 1.8

Objective 1.5: *Given an imaging study, identify processes, technologies, and patient positions used in that study.*

Objective 1.6: *Given an imaging study, identify common contrast media used in that study.*

Objective 1.7: *Given imaging study results or values, identify the associated disease or diagnosis, or given a disease or diagnosis, identify the associated imaging study results or values.*

Objective 1.8: *Given unique imaging study values, identify the correct expression or definition of the values.*

Rationale

Building on the knowledge acquired as one of the basics of medical transcription education, the Level 2 transcriptionist has gained through experience a more comprehensive understanding about a broad range of imaging studies, particularly as such studies are used in acute-care medicine, including the correct expression of relevant terminology. As with the domain of laboratory testing, the experienced acute-care medical transcriptionist also understands the underlying meaning of imaging procedures and results, and will be able to relate specific study protocols, procedures, and results to specific diseases, conditions, and diagnoses. This is a dynamic area, with new technologies appearing frequently, and the medical transcriptionist must be sure to have current and reliable information about the evolution of this branch of clinical medicine diagnostics and treatment.

Recommendations for Focused Study

1. *The Book of Style for Medical Transcription, Third Edition*, Chapters 14-24.
2. *Laboratory Tests and Diagnostic Procedures in Medicine*, J. H. Dirckx (Health Professions Institute)
3. *Human Diseases, Third Edition*, J. H. Dirckx (Health Professions Institute)

Sample Questions

Each question below represents the kind of format and content, per the exam blue print, that a CMT candidate can expect to find on the CMT exam. *Note: These are sample questions only. They are questions that do not currently appear on the CMT exam. Though some may represent items retired from previous exam forms, not all items have been psychometrically analyzed, and AHDI cautions candidates against the presumption that these items alone may be diagnostic or indicative of candidate performance.* (**Answer key at end of chapter.)**

7. What is the procedure for a hysterosalpingogram?

   A. A tube with a balloon is passed through the cervix into the uterus and dye is injected.
   B. A tube with a balloon is placed into the uterus through a tiny pelvic incision and dye is injected.
   C. Radiopaque dye is administered orally and an x-ray view of the pelvis is taken.
   D. Radiopaque dye is administered and a pelvic ultrasound is performed.

8. What procedure inserts a catheter percutaneously and uses an attached balloon to crush an obstruction?

   A. DSA
   B. IVP
   C. PTCA
   D. PTHC

9. What contrast medium is used in MRI studies?

   A. radionuclide
   B. technetium
   C. gadolinium
   D. thallium

10. What medium is used in performing a pulmonary ventilation scan?

   A. radioactive Xe-133
   B. iodine

C. carbon-14
D. pure oxygen

11. What diagnosis does a positive fluorescent ANA suggest?

A. presence of lupus
B. absence of lupus
C. absence of folliculitis
D. presence of acute nephritis

12. A patient's dizziness might be evaluated with what testing?

A. indocyanine green angiogram
B. radioactive uptake iodine test
C. Coombs test
D. electronystagmography

13. What is the correct expression of a measurement based on the rate of decay of a radioactive substance?

A. MCI
B. µMCI
C. mCi
D. MgC

14. Which is the correct expression of a measurement commonly encountered in carotid angiograms?

A. 4F
B. 4 French
C. 4f
D. 4 Fr

Sample Questions Answer Key

1. A
2. A
3. C
4. B
5. D
6. B
7. A
8. C
9. C
10. A
11. A
12. D
13. C
14. B

Anatomy and Physiology
Beyond the Basics

Certified Medical Transcriptionist

Chapter 3

EXAM BLUE PRINT

"Professional Level 2: An incumbent in this position is given assignments that require a seasoned depth of knowledge in a medical specialty (or specialties). OR The incumbent is regularly given assignments that vary in report or correspondence type, originator, and specialty. Incumbents at this level are able to resolve non-routine problems independently, or to assist in resolving complex or highly unusual problems."

– **Medical Transcription Job Descriptions**

Chapter Overview

The expectation that the Level 2 medical transcriptionist will be able to exercise judgment in a variety of specialty contexts implies an active, increasingly in-depth understanding of human anatomy and physiology. For example, acute-care practitioners are often involved in the creation of surgical documentation, and the ability to comprehend surgical processes (particularly in the face of poor dictation habits, less-than perfect English dictation, and complexity of care) is built upon solid anatomical knowledge. Equally, as the complexity of medical contexts increases at the acute-care level, again the exercise of judgment and the resolution of problems are based upon a store of knowledge about human physiological processes that are encountered in clinical medicine in a range of specialties. In other words, a passive ability to understand what a clear and organized speaker says is even less sufficient at this level than it was for the Level 1 practitioner, given the increasing breadth and complexity of medical care that the Level 2 practitioner encounters.

The body of knowledge in anatomy and physiology for the Level 2, acute-care medical transcriptionists therefore includes an understanding of:

- The appearance and position of anatomic features of the human body.
- The positional relationships among anatomic structures, particularly those encountered in surgical practice.
- The processes and functions of human physiology as they are encountered in a variety of clinical specialties and practice.

There are **3 objectives** on the CMT blue print that address concepts related to these domains and against which a CMT exam candidate will be evaluated. In this chapter, we will walk through each objective listed under *CMT Blue Print Section 1: Clinical Medicine* that relate to these domains.

Objective 1.13

Objective 1.13: *Given a graphic showing anatomy or systems, identify the anatomy or system.*

Rationale

The experienced acute-care medical transcriptionist has a cognitive storehouse of mental images and memories related to the structure of the human body. Scientists tell us that storage of these long-term memories is a complex process in the brain involving the manufacture of proteins and the action of the hippocampus. In practical terms, the practitioner needs to possess such images and memories and to be able to call on them when needed; for example, in the midst of a complicated and less than perfectly clear operative report dictation. Many transcriptionists find that being able to summon up a mental image of a procedure greatly assists them in creating an accurate record of that procedure. In any area of clinical practice, these mental images form part of the fund of knowledge that the Level 2 transcriptionist brings to the healthcare documentation process.

Recommendations for Focused Study

1. The US National Library of Medicine and the National Institutes of Health offer free video records of surgical procedures, and there is no better tool for enhancing your understanding of human anatomy as the surgeon and other

healthcare providers see it:
http://www.nlm.nih.gov/medlineplus/surgeryvideos.html

2. *Principles of Human Anatomy, 12th Edition,* G. J. Tortora and M. T. Nielsen (John Wiley and Sons, Inc.)
3. *Human Diseases, 3rd Edition*, J. H. Dirckx, MD (Health Professions Institute)

Sample Questions

Each question below represents the kind of format and content, per the exam blue print, that a CMT candidate can expect to find on the CMT exam. *Note: These are sample questions only. They are questions that do not currently appear on the CMT exam. Though some may represent items retired from previous exam forms, not all items have been psychometrically analyzed, and AHDI cautions candidates against the presumption that these items alone may be diagnostic or indicative of candidate performance.* **(Answer key at end of chapter.)**

1. In the illustration below, what muscle is indicated by the arrow?

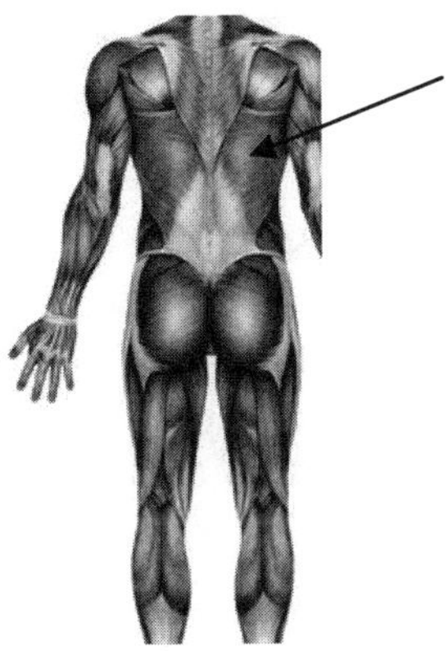

A. infraspinatus
B. latissimus dorsi
C. adductor magnus
D. gluteus medius

2. In the illustration below, what is the name of the muscle the arrow is pointing to?

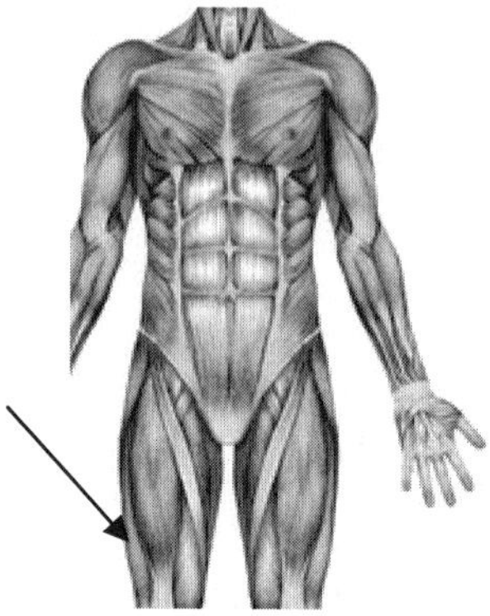

A. vastus lateralis
B. gastrocnemius
C. psoas major
D. soleus

3. What is the name of the bone indicated by the arrow below?

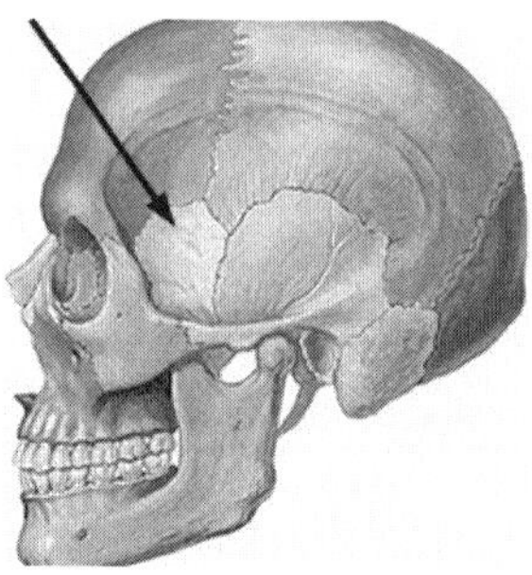

A. occipital
B. parietal
C. frontal
D. sphenoid

Objective 1.14

Objective 1.14: *Given a position or location, identify the anatomical part of the human body.*

Rationale

In anatomical terminology, as in real estate, a critical factor is location, location, location. Common carotid artery, common femoral artery: what difference does it make? Transcriptionists know that the differences may be too numerous to count! In terms of documentation accuracy, patient care, risk management, data analysis, coding, and reimbursement, for example, there's no room for confusing these two terms. And yet it can happen that a surgeon operating in the neck may mention encountering the common femoral artery. The experienced transcriptionist knows that such absent-minded misstatements do occur, and one as obvious as this will ring a very loud bell. There will be other, more subtle misstatements or unclear verbiage which, if perpetuated in an electronic record, may cause considerable subsequent difficulties for all the users of that record: patients, healthcare providers, insurers, data abstractors, and others. The Level 2 practitioner approaching the transcription or editing of any report immediately, without conscious effort, brings into mind the anatomical structures involved, and with that mental picture comes the appropriate vocabulary, not necessarily at the level of conscious thought but as part of the practitioner's fund of knowledge.

Recommendations for Focused Study

1. *Principles of Human Anatomy, 12th Edition,* G. J. Tortora and M. T. Nielsen (John Wiley and Sons, Inc.)
2. *Human Diseases, 3rd Edition,* J. H. Dirckx, MD (Health Professions Institute)

Sample Questions

Each question below represents the kind of format and content, per the exam blue print, that a CMT candidate can expect to find on the CMT exam. *Note: These are sample questions only. They are questions that do not currently appear on the CMT exam. Though some may represent items retired from previous exam forms, not all items have been psychometrically analyzed, and AHDI cautions candidates against the presumption that these items alone may be diagnostic or indicative of candidate performance.* **(Answer key at end of chapter.)**

4. Which ligament runs on the outside of the knee and limits side-to-side motion?

    A. anterior cruciate
    B. lateral collateral
    C. posterior cruciate
    D. medial collateral

5. What is the name of the sac located on the undersurface of the liver?

    A. pancreas
    B. gallbladder
    C. appendix
    D. duodenum

6. What is the small locus of modified cardiac muscle fibers located near the ostium of the coronary sinus that passes impulses toward the ventricle?

    A. Purkinje fibers
    B. sinoatrial node
    C. bundle of His
    D. atrioventricular node

7. What is located at the upper left portion of the abdomen and is the largest of the lymphoid organs?

    A. thymus
    B. spleen
    C. liver
    D. gallbladder

Objective 1.15

Objective 1.15: *Given a physiologic process, identify the steps or functions related to that process.*

Rationale

The complex functions of the human body begin at the level of atoms (such as oxygen) and molecules (such as DNA), and operate within the tissues, organs, and organ systems of the body. For the most part, clinical dictation will be concerned with the tissue, organ, and organ-system levels of these processes, though some basic background understanding of the atomic and molecular levels can be useful for medical transcriptionists as well. The acute-care, experienced transcriptionist encounters physiologic functions and their attendant terminologies in the context of various medical specialties; each level of function has its own unique vocabulary, and this vocabulary is augmented and focused by the concerns of the specialty involved. No one practitioner can be totally cognizant of all these terminologies, but with increasing depth and breadth of experience, the Level 2 transcriptionist accumulates increasing depth and breadth of knowledge. That process of the accumulation of knowledge mirrors, in a sense, the healthy physiological functions of the body, each step building on the steps that came before, and contributing ultimately to the healthy life of the whole organism or, in the case of the medical transcription function, to an accurate and complete healthcare document.

Recommendations for Focused Study

1. *Principles of Human Anatomy, 12th Edition,* G. J. Tortora and M. T. Nielsen (John Wiley and Sons, Inc.)
2. *Human Diseases, 3rd Edition*, J. H. Dirckx, MD (Health Professions Institute)

Sample Questions

Each question below represents the kind of format and content, per the exam blue print, that a CMT candidate can expect to find on the CMT exam. *Note: These are sample questions only. They are questions that do not currently appear on the CMT exam. Though some may represent items retired from previous exam forms, not all items have been psychometrically analyzed, and AHDI cautions candidates against the presumption that these items alone may be diagnostic or indicative of candidate performance.* **(Answer key at end of chapter.)**

8. Glomerular filtration, tubular reabsorption, and tubular secretion are involved in what physiologic process?

   A. urine production
   B. respiration
   C. metabolic glucose cycle
   D. production of thyroid hormones

9. Choose the correct pathway for inhaled air.

   A. pharynx, trachea, larynx, bronchi, bronchioles, lung capillaries, alveoli
   B. pharynx, larynx, trachea, bronchi, bronchioles, alveoli, lung capillaries
   C. larynx, pharynx, trachea, bronchi, bronchioles, alveoli, lung capillaries
   D. pharynx, larynx, trachea, bronchioles, bronchi, lung capillaries, alveoli

10. What describes part of the process in which blood glucose levels are regulated?

    A. The anterior lobe of the pituitary produces insulin and the posterior lobe produces glucagon.
    B. The adrenal medulla secretes epinephrine and norepinephrine.
    C. The pancreatic islets produce insulin and glucagon.
    D. The pancreatic islets secrete epinephrine and norepinephrine.

Sample Questions Answer Key

1. B
2. A
3. D
4. B
5. B
6. D
7. B
8. A
9. B
10. C

Understanding Clinical Practice

Certified Medical Transcriptionist

Chapter 4

EXAM BLUE PRINT

"If some transcriptionists now have less keystroking to perform, their editorial function has expanded as they are challenged to correct not only dictators' errors of commission and omission, but also those perpetrated by the machinery."

– John H. Dirckx, MD. "Foreword," *The Book of Style for Medical Transcription, 3rd Edition.*

Chapter Overview

The Level 2 acute-care medical transcriptionist, with two or more years of documentation experience, has advanced beyond a thorough understanding of the basic terminologies and concepts of clinical practice. At this level, the transcriptionist will possess advanced knowledge in multiple medical specialties and will be able to exercise judgment in the creation of the healthcare document, encompassing not only office-based or clinic-based medicine but also medicine as practiced in major hospitals and tertiary-care centers. The acute-care transcriptionist has a broad understanding of the diagnosis, classification, and treatment of disease. Arguably, the knowledge the acute-care transcriptionist brings to documentation has become even more crucial with increasing adoption of speech recognition and related technologies. The Level 2 medical transcriptionist will be able to reliably decipher (or know when to query) unclear or ambivalent dictation or data entry, will not be confused by errors in SR transcription or other automated systems, and will be a major contributor to documentation accuracy.

The body of knowledge about clinical practice for Level 2 medical transcriptionists therefore includes an understanding of:

- Signs and symptoms of diseases and syndromes.
- Standard treatment courses.
- Uses of medications in specific diseases and conditions.
- The complex relationships among signs and symptoms, exam findings, diagnostic testing results, and diagnoses for a broad spectrum of diseases and conditions.
- The meanings and applications of classification systems for a broad spectrum of diseases and conditions.

There are **6 objectives**[1] on the CMT blue print that address concepts related to these domains and against which a CMT exam candidate will be evaluated. In this chapter, we will walk through each objective listed under *CMT Blue Print Section 1: Clinical Medicine* that relate to these domains.

Objective 1.16

Objective 1.16: *Given a sign or symptom, identify the disease or syndrome, or given a disease or syndrome, identify the sign or symptom.*

Rationale

To the task of either transcribing dictation or editing voice-recognized files, the acute-care transcriptionist brings a depth of knowledge about signs and symptoms associated with specific diseases and syndromes. This knowledge provides a timely quality assessment at the point of creation of a healthcare document. This function may prove particularly valuable in monitoring the accuracy of records created with point-and-click, drop-down menus, or other technologies that may increase the possibility of error.

---

[1] Objectives 1.20 and 1.28 on the CMT blue print are audio objectives that also relate to Understanding Clinical Practice. Look for blue print guidance on audio objectives in upcoming AHDI exam prep products.

Recommendations for Focused Study

1. *Book of Style for Medical Transcription, Third Edition*, Section 4.
2. *"Profiles of Common Medical Conditions," Stedman's Medical Dictionary for the Health Professions and Nursing, Illustrated 6th Edition,* pp. APP 263-APP 273.
3. *Principles of Human Anatomy, 12th Edition*, Tortora and Nielsen, (John Wiley and Sons, Inc.: "Clinical Connections" (see Table of Contents, pp. xxvi-xxvii).

Sample Questions

Each question below represents the kind of format and content, per the exam blue print, that a CMT candidate can expect to find on the CMT exam. *Note: These are sample questions only. They are questions that do not currently appear on the CMT exam. Though some may represent items retired from previous exam forms, not all items have been psychometrically analyzed, and AHDI cautions candidates against the presumption that these items alone may be diagnostic or indicative of candidate performance.* **(Answer key at end of chapter.)**

1. Barrett esophagus is a possible complication in patients with what diagnosis?

    A. TMJ
    B. GERD
    C. EBV
    D. ESRD

2. Pain and paresthesias in the thumb and index finger, especially at night, are symptoms of what condition?

    A. rheumatoid arthritis
    B. Colles fracture
    C. carpal tunnel syndrome
    D. Dupuytren contracture

Objective 1.17

Objective 1.17: *Given a disease or syndrome, identify the treatment course.*

Rationale

The experienced acute-care medical transcriptionist brings to the healthcare documentation process an ability to anticipate (though not assume) correct text, whether dictated or created by speech recognition. Knowledge of standard treatment courses for a variety of diseases and syndromes is one of the central elements of accurate transcription and editing, allowing the transcriptionist to not only reliably interpret unclear dictation or inaccurate voice recognition but to also recognize errors or ambiguities that require additional input from the record originator.

Recommendations for Focused Study

1. *"*Profiles of Common Medical Conditions,*" Stedman's Medical Dictionary for the Health Professions and Nursing, Illustrated 6th Edition*, pp. APP 263-APP 273.
2. *Case Files® Surgery, Third Edition*, Toy, Liu, and Campbell (McGraw Hill Medical)

Sample Questions

Each question below represents the kind of format and content, per the exam blue print, that a CMT candidate can expect to find on the CMT exam. *Note: These are sample questions only. They are questions that do not currently appear on the CMT exam. Though some may represent items retired from previous exam forms, not all items have been psychometrically analyzed, and AHDI cautions candidates against the presumption that these items alone may be diagnostic or indicative of candidate performance.* (**Answer key at end of chapter.)**

3. What would be a treatment course for acute pancreatitis?

   A. emergency laparotomy
   B. tube feeding with fluid restriction, modified bed rest
   C. bed rest and modified diet
   D. fluid resuscitation, pain management

4. What would be a recommended course of treatment for plantar fasciitis?

   A. casting and long-term antibiotics
   B. stretching exercises and anti-inflammatories

C. outpatient surgery followed by antibiotics
D. outpatient surgery followed by casting

Objective 1.21

Objective 1.21: *Given a medication, identify the symptom or disease for which it is prescribed, or given a symptom or disease, identify the medication that is prescribed.*

Rationale

The entry-level Registered Medical Transcriptionist came to the profession armed with a basic knowledge of pharmacology, including the functions, administration, and categories of medications. The acute-care Certified Medical Transcriptionist then builds on these basics and adds extensive knowledge about the uses of specific medications in a variety of specialties for treatment of disease and symptoms.

Recommendations for Focused Study

1. *Quick Look Drug Book 2011*, Lippincott, Williams, and Wilkins.
2. *Saunders Pharmaceutical Word Book 2011,* Drake and Drake

Sample Questions

Each question below represents the kind of format and content, per the exam blue print, that a CMT candidate can expect to find on the CMT exam. *Note: These are sample questions only. They are questions that do not currently appear on the CMT exam. Though some may represent items retired from previous exam forms, not all items have been psychometrically analyzed, and AHDI cautions candidates against the presumption that these items alone may be diagnostic or indicative of candidate performance.* (**Answer key at end of chapter.)**

5. What condition would be treated with a prescription for the topical retinoid tazarotene?

   A. Crohn disease
   B. candidiasis
   C. pediculosis capitis
   D. psoriasis

6. What medication would be used in the treatment of Lyme disease?

A. doxycycline
B. aripiprazole
C. olmesartan
D. omeprazole

Objective 1.22

Objective 1.22: *Given a diagnostic scenario that could include signs/symptoms, physical exam findings, diagnostic test results, and diagnosis, identify information about the signs/symptoms, physical exam findings, diagnostics test results, and diagnosis.*

Rationale

The acute-care medical transcriptionist brings to healthcare documentation an understanding of the complete picture of clinical practice. This understanding encompasses the signs and symptoms and physical findings of a patient's initial encounter with healthcare providers, proceeding through the diagnostic process including imaging and laboratory testing, to the patient's ultimate diagnosis. While each patient is unique, the acute-care transcriptionist is familiar with a range of more or less commonly occurring scenarios, and applies that knowledge to the creation of an accurate, coherent healthcare document.

Recommendations for Focused Study

1. "Profiles of Common Medical Conditions," *Stedman's Medical Dictionary for the Health Professions and Nursing, Illustrated 6th Edition*, pp. APP 263-APP 273.
2. *Case Files® Surgery, Third Edition,* , Toy, Liu, and Campbell (McGraw Hill Medical)
3. *Principles of Human Anatomy, 12th Edition (Tortora and Nielsen)*: "Clinical Connections" (see Table of Contents, pp. xxvi-xxvii).

Sample Questions

Each question below represents the kind of format and content, per the exam blue print, that a CMT candidate can expect to find on the CMT exam. *Note: These are sample questions only. They are questions that do not currently appear on the CMT exam. Though some may represent items retired from previous exam forms, not all items have been psychometrically analyzed, and AHDI cautions candidates against the presumption that these items alone may be diagnostic or indicative of candidate performance.* (**Answer key at end of chapter.)**

7. **A(n) _________ will be ordered as an initial diagnostic step in evaluation of this patient's dominant thyroid nodule.**

   What kind of test or exam is most likely to be performed?

   A. plain x-ray
   B. scintigraphy
   C. fine-needle aspiration biopsy
   D. PET scan

8. **A postoperative patient is noted in the recovery room to have indicators of volume depletion including __________ and ___________.**

   What are the likely signs or symptoms mentioned in the blanks?

   A. hypertension and excessive urine output
   B. hypotension and excessive urine output
   C. hypotension and low urine output
   D. hypertension and low urine output

9. **Several weeks following the onset of pancreatitis, the patient developed an accumulation of thick, purulent fluid, as seen on MRI scan, with an elevated white count and was diagnosed with __________, for which surgery was recommended and performed.**

   What was the diagnosis in the above scenario?

   A. severe biliary stenosis
   B. pancreatic abscess

C. biliary tract carcinoma
D. pancreatic carcinoma

Objectives 1.23 and 1.24

Objective 1.23: *Given a classification system, identify the expressed score or grade.*

Objective 1.24: *Given a classification system result, identify the disease or affected anatomical part.*

Rationale

Classification systems in the practice of medicine provide a means of succinct but specific communication among healthcare providers, researchers, and patients. At the point of creation of the clinical document, the experienced medical transcriptionist/editor can contribute to clarity and integrity by ensuring that classifications are presented in a consistent manner and are appropriate for the clinical context. Each specialty and aspect of medical practice has a unique set of classification systems; at the acute-care level, the transcriptionist is familiar with the details of a broad range of these systems.

Recommendations for Focused Study

The Book of Style for Medical Transcription, Third Edition, Sections 14.3, 16.2.1, 16.2.2, 17.1.3, 18.1.5, 18.2.4, 19.1.4, 19.2.3, 20.3, 22.2, 23.3, and 24.2

Sample Questions

Each question below represents the kind of format and content, per the exam blue print, that a CMT candidate can expect to find on the CMT exam. *Note: These are sample questions only. They are questions that do not currently appear on the CMT exam. Though some may represent items retired from previous exam forms, not all items have been psychometrically analyzed, and AHDI cautions candidates against the presumption that these items alone may be diagnostic or indicative of candidate performance.* **(Answer key at end of chapter.)**

10. Which is a finding in the Bethesda classification system?

A. ASCUS
B. MEN 2A
C. LUAVPG
D. CD3d

11. A child diagnosed with a crush injury to the physis would be classified how?

A. LeFort I
B. Rancho Los Amigos VI
C. Mayo IIIA
D. Salter-Harris V

12. **On physical examination we found asymmetry, irregularity, color variation, and a 3 cm diameter.**

What is being evaluated?

A. a burned area of skin surface
B. the iris of the eye
C. a lesion suspicious for melanoma
D. sclerodermatous skin changes

13. What condition is being described when a patient is classified as Dukes B?

A. malignant melanoma
B. leukemia
C. colon carcinoma
D. lymphoma

Sample Questions Answer Key

1. B
2. C
3. D
4. B
5. D
6. A
7. C
8. C
9. B
10. A
11. D
12. C
13. C

Understanding Surgical Practice

Certified Medical Transcriptionist
Chapter 5
EXAM BLUE PRINT

"While transcriptionists do not provide hands-on patient care, they are part of a critical process to create an accurate record of that care and, if unprepared, carry the potential for adversely affecting that process and/or hindering operational efficiency."

– **AHDI Credentialing Candidate Guide**

Chapter Overview

If it can be said that there is one area of medicine that defines the acute-care medical transcriptionist, that area would be surgical practice. While the entry-level transcriptionist is expected to have knowledge about the basic terminology and procedures of surgery, the Level 2 medical transcriptionist will have added to that basic knowledge a sophisticated understanding of how and why surgeries are performed, including techniques in a range of surgical specialties, along with the attendant procedures, equipment, and standards of practice. Further, the Level 2 transcriptionist will be prepared to bring a seasoned depth of knowledge and analytical focus to bear on complex issues concerning the accuracy and integrity of the healthcare document. Nowhere are accuracy and integrity more important than in the documentation surrounding surgical practice. The ability of the CMT to understand, interpret, and assess quality in complex surgical dictation, often from authors speaking heavily accented or imperfect English, as well as in speech-recognized documents, is the hallmark of the experienced Level 2 medical transcription practitioner.

The body of knowledge for acute-care medical transcriptionists in the domain of surgical practice therefore includes an understanding of:

- Standard surgical approaches and techniques associated with specific procedures in a wide variety of specialties.
- Equipment and instruments associated with specific kinds of surgical procedures.
- A thorough knowledge of specialty-specific language commonly used in descriptions of surgical procedures, approaches, and techniques.

There are **3 objectives** on the CMT blue print that address concepts related to this domain and against which a CMT exam candidate will be evaluated. In this chapter, we will walk through each objective listed under *CMT Blue Print Section 1: Clinical Medicine* that relate to surgical practice.

Objective 1.25

Objective 1.25: *Given a surgical approach or technique (anesthesia, positions, incisions, suture techniques, etc.), identify the procedure with which it is associated.*

Rationale

Interpretation and correct transcription or editing of surgical documents requires more than a passive understanding of terminology. The skill set brought to this documentation process by the experienced medical transcriptionist/editor is strengthened by an understanding of the relationship between given approaches or techniques and specific kinds of surgical procedures. This will include all the elements involved in performance of surgery: administration of and types of anesthesia commonly used; positioning of patients for specific procedures; kinds of incisions and suture types and techniques employed in the approach to specific surgeries; and any other aspects of a given surgery. This understanding supports the function of the transcriptionist as an assessor of document quality at the moment of document creation, so that unclear or mistaken dictation or speech-recognized text can be corrected or flagged for the healthcare provider's review.

Recommendations for Focused Study

The CMT Review Guide (Stedman's); Chapters 4 through 25.

Sample Questions

Each question below represents the kind of format and content, per the exam blue print, that a CMT candidate can expect to find on the CMT exam. *Note: These are sample questions only. They are questions that do not currently appear on the CMT exam. Though some may represent items retired from previous exam forms, not all items have been psychometrically analyzed, and AHDI cautions candidates against the presumption that these items alone may be diagnostic or indicative of candidate performance.* **(Answer key at end of chapter.)**

1. What type of procedure involves a low transverse abdominal incision?

   A. open appendectomy
   B. primary cesarean section
   C. colonoscopy
   D. Whipple procedure

2. The Roux-en-Y technique is used in which kind of surgical specialty?

   A. bariatric
   B. arthroscopic
   C. urologic
   D. ophthalmologic

3. What kind of surgery uses an anterior approach through the sternocleidomastoid muscle?

   A. inguinal hernia repair
   B. cervical diskectomy
   C. SLAP repair
   D. lumbar fusion

Objective 1.26

Objective 1.26: *Given surgical equipment or a surgical instrument, identify the procedure with which it is associated.*

Rationale

The domain of surgical devices offers a particular challenge to the acute-care medical transcriptionist. As is the case with new drugs, new equipment and new instruments for surgery are constantly being developed and introduced into surgical practice. Other factors complicate the transcriptionist/editor's work to produce accurate records of surgical procedures. One is that instruments commonly used in one type of procedure may, in the hands of a specific surgeon, be used in a different type of procedure. Another, though less common, occurrence is that a surgeon may develop and use unique instruments (sometimes bearing the surgeon's own name) that are not in widespread use outside of that local practice or region. Here, as is true in other realms of medical transcription and editing, experience with particular clinicians is of great value. At the same time, the Level 2 transcriptionist will have at his or her own fingertips an extensive lexicon of terms for surgical procedures in a variety of specialties, and use this knowledge to avoid ambiguities or errors in operative reports.

Recommendations for Focused Study

The CMT Review Guide (Stedman's); Chapters 4 through 25.

Sample Questions

Each question below represents the kind of format and content, per the exam blue print, that a CMT candidate can expect to find on the CMT exam. *Note: These are sample questions only. They are questions that do not currently appear on the CMT exam. Though some may represent items retired from previous exam forms, not all items have been psychometrically analyzed, and AHDI cautions candidates against the presumption that these items alone may be diagnostic or indicative of candidate performance.* (**Answer key at end of chapter.**)

4. What procedure would use a #2 cutting block?

A. appendectomy
B. total knee arthroplasty
C. rhinoplasty
D. arteriotomy
A.

5. During what procedure would a pigtail catheter be used?

A. cystectomy
B. left heart catheterization
C. oophorectomy
D. prostatectomy

6. A Mayfield holder would be used in what type of surgery?

A. abdominal
B. thoracic
C. cardiac
D. cranial

7. In which type of surgery might a peel-away sheath be used?

A. repair of an AVM
B. FNA of the breast
C. implantation of an AICD
D. implantation of an IOL

Objective 1.27

Objective 1.27: *Given an excerpt from an operative report, identify the procedure that was conducted.*

Rationale

The experienced acute-care transcriptionist is an active assessor of healthcare document quality and, therefore, passive acceptance of dictated content, however correctly transcribed, falls short of expectations for medical transcription practitioners at this level. Particularly in a context of templating, drop-down menus, point-and-click entry, and other automated means of creating a healthcare document, the medical transcriptionist/editor must have the ability to identify and query potential inaccuracies in documentation at or near the point of origination of the document. This may be particularly important for the content of operative reports, where missteps in document creation may have major impacts on patient care and safety, and leave healthcare practitioners vulnerable in terms of medicolegal risk.

Recommendations for Focused Study

The CMT Review Guide (Stedman's); Chapters 4 through 25.

Sample Questions

Each question below represents the kind of format and content, per the exam blue print, that a CMT candidate can expect to find on the CMT exam. *Note: These are sample questions only. They are questions that do not currently appear on the CMT exam. Though some may represent items retired from previous exam forms, not all items have been psychometrically analyzed, and AHDI cautions candidates against the presumption that these items alone may be diagnostic or indicative of candidate performance.* (**Answer key at end of chapter.)**

8. **With the patient in the lateral decubitus position and using arthroscopy, sutures were passed through the superior labrum anteriorly and posteriorly.**

   What surgical procedure is being described in the above sentence?

   A. repair of SLAP lesion
   B. repair of patellar tendon
   C. repair of Dupuytren contracture
   D. repair of Sinding-Larsen-Johansson lesion

9. **To allow mobilization of the tissue, the galea was incised in multiple areas, then the tissue was closed with 3-0 Vicryl suture deep in the galea.**

In what kind of surgery would the above sentence be found?

A. Total hip replacement
B. Total knee replacement
C. Scalp tumor resection
D. Resection of renal tumor

10. **Marcaine 2 mL was used on the superficial skin over the A1 pulley.**

In what surgical procedure would the above phrase be found?

A. total knee arthroplasty
B. carpal tunnel release
C. closed ORIF
D. transforaminal neuroplasty

Sample Questions Answer Key

1. B
2. A
3. B
4. B
5. B
6. D
7. C
8. A
9. C
10. B

Section 2

Health Information Technology

"I earned my CMT credential many years ago and have maintained it because it provides me with better paying job opportunities and also provides a sense of self-pride that I can prove I continue to stay involved in my industry."

– Cynthia Alder, CMT, RHIT, AHDI-F

Health IT: Terminology & Fundamentals

Certified Medical Transcriptionist

Chapter 6

EXAM BLUE PRINT

"Transcribed reports are only part of the patient's record. The final product of an MT's effort must meld into the bigger healthcare documentation picture. As more and more of the healthcare industry embraces information technology, we too must learn these technologies in order to work in tandem with health information technicians and administrators."

– **Technology for the Medical Transcriptionist**[1]

Chapter Overview

A significant challenge for the clinical documentation sector will be forecasting both the rate of EHR adoption nationwide and the degree to which healthcare documentation roles will evolve and change as a result of this technology. While some things cannot be predicted, most experts agree that the demand for data integrity will only increase, creating an opportunity for the risk management skill set of the medical transcriptionist. AHDI and its allied partners continue to advocate for the tacit knowledge of our workforce and the value that an interpretive knowledge worker can offer in tandem with these enabling technologies. An accurate, complete health record that can be securely stored, accessed, and repurposed within an interoperable delivery system is healthcare's primary goal for EHRs, and the MT who

---

[1] Bryan, Laura MT (ASCP), CMT, AHDI-F. *Technology for the Medical Transcriptionist.* Baltimore: Wolters Kluwer, 2010.

understands the technology and its objectives can help facilitate high-integrity adoption and integration as well as continue to be an evolving, contributory player in health data capture and documentation. This means the advanced, Level 2 documentation specialist needs to understand more than just how these technologies work. MTs also need to understand the definitions, criteria, standards, and codified languages that have been created around the use and integration of EHR systems.

The body of knowledge for Level 2 medical transcriptionists in this domain therefore includes an understanding of:

- Health IT standards and standards-setting organizations, both by name and abbreviation/acronym.
- Terminology and definitions related to EHR systems, adoption, and integration.
- Regulatory terms and definitions related to EHR adoption.
- Clinical nomenclature and coding systems that are used in health information management, narrative capture, and data abstracting.

There are **4 objectives** on the CMT blue print that address concepts related to these domains and against which a CMT exam candidate will be evaluated. In this chapter, we will walk through each objective listed under *CMT Blue Print Section 2: Health Information Technology* that relate to these domains.

Objectives 2.1 and 2.2

Objective 2.1: *Given an abbreviation, identify the correctly expanded form.*

Objective 2.2: *Given an EHR technology term, identify the correct definition, or given a definition, identify the correct EHR technology term.*

Rationale

Nationwide EHR adoption is now an inevitability, not just a possibility. All health information, regardless of how or by whom it is captured and documented, will have to integrate into the EHR systems of today and the future. This means that traditional transcription in an isolated word processing environment will likely give way to systems and standards that drive how free text narrative is formatted and codified for export and consumption in those EHR systems. A Level 2 MT needs to be well informed and ready to adapt to changing systems and integration requirements. This has to start with a foundational understanding of EHR systems, terms, and abbreviations, as well as the organizations responsible for setting those standards and definitions.

Recommendations for Focused Study

1. *EHR Glossary* – Included in Appendix D
2. *Technology for the Medical Transcriptionist*, Bryan (Wolters Kluwer Health/Lippincott Williams and Wilkins) Transcription Technology, Chapter 15 (The Electronic Health Record, pp 524-534).
3. *EHR Readiness Tool Kit* (AHDI)
   www.ahdionline.org – Professional Practices/Tool Kits/EHR Readiness
4. *The Book of Style for Medical Transcription,* 3rd Edition (AHDI)
   Chapters 25 and 26.[2]

Sample Questions

Each question below represents the kind of format and content, per the exam blue print, that a CMT candidate can expect to find on the CMT exam. *Note: These are sample questions only. They are questions that do not currently appear on the CMT exam. Though some may represent items retired from previous exam forms, not all items have been psychometrically analyzed, and AHDI cautions candidates against the presumption that these items alone may be diagnostic or indicative of candidate performance.* **(Answer key at end of chapter.)**

---

[2] *Note:* CDA4CDT, identified and discussed in Chapter 26 of the 3rd edition Book of Style, has since been renamed *The Health Story Project,* and any questions related to this organization that are found in this text or on the AHDI CMT exam are based on this new identification.

1. Which organization sets standards for interoperability and publishes specifications/protocols used by software developers who create interfaces between health IT computer systems?

   A. SNOMED
   B. AMA
   C. HL7
   D. CDA

2. Which refers to the process of gathering and storing information from patient progress notes, imaging reports, transcribed notes, and other clinical sources into a single healthcare record?

   A. documentation
   B. data capture
   C. record keeping
   D. interoperability

3. What does the "M" in *ASTM* refer to?

   A. materials
   B. management
   C. medicine
   D. manual

4. Which is a delayed data capture method that is not performed in "real time" at the point of care?

   A. Dictation/transcription
   B. Point-and-click template systems
   C. Front-end speech recognition
   D. Radiofrequency identification

5. Which organization, established by the Office of the National Coordinator for Health IT, certifies the *products* that meet or exceed standards for usability and interoperability?

   A. HL7
   B. HITSP
   C. CCHIT
   D. RHIO

Objectives 2.7 and 2.8

Objective 2.7: *Given a term or concept related to nomenclatures or measurement systems, identify the correct definition.*

Objective 2.8: *Given a term or concept related to NLP, identify the correct definition.*

Rationale

As healthcare delivery migrates from an ICD-9 to an ICD-10 coding system and regulatory standards for reimbursement continue to shape the way health encounters are documented, it will become increasingly more important for all members of the health information management, including MTs, to understand what these requirements and standards are.

Recommendations for Focused Study

1. *Technology for the Medical Transcriptionist*, Bryan (Wolters Kluwer Health/Lippincott Williams and Wilkins)
   Transcription Technology, Chapter 15
2. *The Book of Style for Medical Transcription,* 3rd Edition (AHDI)
   Chapter 27: Systematized Nomenclature for Medicine (SNOMED)

Sample Questions

Each question below represents the kind of format and content, per the exam blue print, that a CMT candidate can expect to find on the CMT exam. *Note: These are sample questions only. They are questions that do not currently appear on the CMT exam. Though some may represent items retired from previous exam forms, not all items have been psychometrically analyzed, and AHDI cautions candidates against the presumption that these items alone may be diagnostic or indicative of candidate performance.* **(Answer key at end of chapter.)**

6. Which abbreviation refers to an enforced audit being mandated by the Centers for Medicare and Medicaid (CMS) to review improper payments made to healthcare providers?

   A. MAC
   B. PQRI
   C. RAC
   D. P4P

7. The Centers for Medicare and Medicaid have worked in collaboration with The Joint Commission to develop a requirement that hospitals collect evidence-based data on certain identified conditions and treatment programs. What is this set of required care processes called?

   A. core measures
   B. meaningful use
   C. pay for performance
   D. data analytics

8. What is SNOMED?

   A. clinical nomenclature system
   B. computer-suggested coding program
   C. integrated data management platform
   D. performance measurement standard

9. Natural language processing is also referred to as natural language ______________.

A. interpretation
B. recognition
C. understanding
D. management

10. What is the primary function of NLP technology?

A. To capture dictated narrative and create a speech-recognized draft.
B. To enable disparate health IT systems to exchange data.
C. To format narrative reports in compliance with HL7's CDA standards.
D. To codify unstructured narrative against data measurement systems for electronic use and analysis.

Sample Questions Answer Key

1. C
2. B
3. A
4. A
5. C
6. C
7. A
8. A
9. C
10. D

Speech Recognition Technology & Practice

Certified Medical Transcriptionist
Chapter 7
EXAM BLUE PRINT

"If some transcriptionists now have less keystroking to perform, their editorial function has expanded as they are challenged to correct not only dictators' errors of commission and omission, but also those perpetrated by the machinery."

– John H. Dirckx, MD. "Foreword," *The Book of Style for Medical Transcription, 3rd Edition*[1]

Chapter Overview

As our society continues to move toward healthcare's vision for a national health information network, the need for digital methods of dictation/transcription grows, and the use of back-end speech recognition technology (SRT) continues to gain momentum in replacing traditional transcription. Within this process, we have seen how the role of medical transcriptionist has changed to that of SRT editor. In order to be an effective SRT editor, it takes the medical knowledge, training, and an eye for detail that MTs already possess, but it also takes enhanced critical thinking skills, focus, and concentration to ensure a quality outcome. While variability of technologies and originator's dictation habits impact the level of accuracy achieved through the process of voice to text, it will be the SRT editor's ability to successfully interpret what the eyes see against what the ears hear and the brain knows that will produce desired results.

---

[1] Sims, Lea M, CMT, AHDI-F. *The Book of Style for Medical Transcription, Third Edition.* Modesto: AHDI, 2008.

The body of knowledge about speech recognition technology and practice for Level 2 medical transcriptionists therefore includes an understanding of:

- Terminology, definitions, abbreviations, and concepts related to speech recognition technology.
- Factors that contribute to or inhibit the successful workflow process of SRT.
- Choosing the correct approach to applying Book of Style standards in SRT.

There are **3 objectives**[2] on the CMT blue print that address concepts related to these domains and against which a CMT exam candidate will be evaluated. In this chapter, we will walk through each objective listed under *CMT Blue Print Section 2: Health Information Technology* that relate to these domains.

Objective 2.3

Objective 2.3: *Given an SRT term or concept, identify the correct definition, or given a definition, identify the correct SRT term or concept.*

Rationale

A skilled medical transcriptionist/SR editor who understands speech recognition terminology and concepts will better be able to adapt to new technologies implemented and recognize, identify, and correct errors produced. While productivity is always on the mind of the MT/SR editor, quality must never be sacrificed for quantity.

Recommendations for Focused Study

1. *The Book of Style for Medical Transcription, 3rd Edition,* Chapter 28: Speech Recognition and SR Editing

[2] Objective 2.6 on the CMT blue print is an audio objective that also relate to Health Information Technology. Look for blue print guidance on audio objectives in upcoming AHDI exam prep products.

2. *Technology for the Medical Transcriptionist*, Bryan (Lippincott Williams & Wilkins)
   Chapter 16: Speech Recognition
3. AHDI/TRSi Speech Recognition Editing Course

Sample Questions

Each question below represents the kind of format and content, per the exam blue print, that a CMT candidate can expect to find on the CMT exam. *Note: These are sample questions only. They are questions that do not currently appear on the CMT exam. Though some may represent items retired from previous exam forms, not all items have been psychometrically analyzed, and AHDI cautions candidates against the presumption that these items alone may be diagnostic or indicative of candidate performance.* **(Answer key at end of chapter.)**

1. Which of the following is a speech recognition technology that uses traditionally recorded voice files?

   A. OAD transcription
   B. natural language processing
   C. front-end SRT
   D. back-end SRT

2. Given a facility's use of voice recognition technology, which of the following may be the responsibility of the documentation specialist (MT)?

   A. draft document editing
   B. real-time correction of draft document
   C. dictation of narrative
   D. authentication of reports

3. Which of the following requires the dictator to edit text as dictation occurs?

   A. front-end speech recognition
   B. natural language processing
   C. back-end speech recognition
   D. all speech recognition engines

4. Front-end SRT may include which of the following?

   A. flagging of report for physician clarification
   B. physician correction of draft document
   C. training the MT to edit
   D. reformatting of reports prior to authentication

5. A rural clinic is comparing costs among SRT vendors. Which of the following may influence the actual return on investment?

   A. number of sales visits per contracted year
   B. projected cost savings as per vendor
   C. ROI of large hospitals in the area
   D. training and implementation costs

Objective 2.4

Objective 2.4: *Given a list, identify success factors for SRT adoption/integration as defined by the Book of Style.*

Rationale

The Level 2 medical transcriptionist/SR editor is a committed member of the healthcare team, bringing life-long learning to the helm when it comes to new technologies, terminology, and techniques. The applied knowledge of the aforementioned along with intense concentration for the task at hand will enhance efficiency and productivity during the SRT integration process.

Recommendations for Focused Study

1. *The Book of Style for Medical Transcription, 3rd Edition*
   Chapter 28: Speech Recognition and SR Editing
2. *Technology for the Medical Transcriptionist*, Bryan (Lippincott Williams & Wilkins)
   Chapter 16: Speech Recognition
3. AHDI/TRSi Speech Recognition Editing Course

Sample Questions

Each question below represents the kind of format and content, per the exam blue print, that a CMT candidate can expect to find on the CMT exam. *Note: These are sample questions only. They are questions that do not currently appear on the CMT exam. Though some may represent items retired from previous exam forms, not all items have been psychometrically analyzed, and AHDI cautions candidates against the presumption that these items alone may be diagnostic or indicative of candidate performance.* (**Answer key at end of chapter.)**

6. According to the Book of Style, what is one of the factors impacting SRT adoption and integration?

   A. dictation habits
   B. federal legislation
   C. type of healthcare facility
   D. range of medical specialties involved

7. Which is a factor impacting SRT adoption and integration?

   A. patient consent
   B. government approval
   C. Joint Commission standards
   D. efficiency and skill set of the editor

8. Which of the following may negatively impact adoption/integration for SRT?

   A. consistent dictator speech patterns
   B. high accuracy of draft documents
   C. hardware/software amortization
   D. low training costs

Objective 2.5

Objective 2.5: *Given scenarios, identify the correct application of Book of Style standards for resolving style conflicts in an SRT editing environment.*

Rationale

While the application of Book of Style standards to speech-recognized documents is not a cut-and-dried process, the decision for an organization to incorporate changes when a style conflict arises may be necessary to maintain the accuracy and integrity of the document. In order to maintain productivity in the speech recognition setting, the Level 2 medical transcriptionist/SR editor must know when to make changes that will enhance clarity of the record and let go some of the non-critical standards that does not compromise quality.

Recommendations for Focused Study

1. *The Book of Style for Medical Transcription, 3rd Edition*
   Chapter 28: Speech Recognition and SR Editing
2. *Technology for the Medical Transcriptionist* (Lippincott Williams and Wilkins)
   Chapter 16: Speech Recognition
3. AHDI/TRSi Speech Recognition Editing Course

Sample Questions

Each question below represents the kind of format and content, per the exam blue print, that a CMT candidate can expect to find on the CMT exam. *Note: These are sample questions only. They are questions that do not currently appear on the CMT exam. Though some may represent items retired from previous exam forms, not all items have been psychometrically analyzed, and AHDI cautions candidates against the presumption that these items alone may be diagnostic or indicative of candidate performance.* (**Answer key at end of chapter.**)

9. An SRT draft document states "no allergies" on page 1 and "allergic to penicillin" on page 3. What step should the editor take?

   A. delete "no allergies" from page 1
   B. leave as originally drafted
   C. listen to voice file
   D. flag for physician to verify

10. A back-end SRT draft document has no blanks when the editor first views it. The next step would be to:

A. spellcheck
B. listen to the audio file
C. verify diagnoses
D. send for physician signature

11. The SRT draft document repeatedly refers to the patient as Charles Smith in the body of the report. This does not match the ADT feed/demographic header of "Casey Smith." What step should the editor take?

A. leave the report as is and send for physician signature
B. change "Charles Smith" to "the patient" throughout the report
C. flag for physician to clarify
D. change demographic header to "Charles Smith"

12. The SRT draft document contains the sentence, "The patient is wide court elevator." On reviewing the audio, the MT editor determines the voice file is inaudible. S/he should:

A. delete the sentence
B. leave the sentence as is, adding [sic] to indicate verbatim
C. edit to "The patient's white count was elevated."
D. flag for clarification

Sample Questions Answer Key

1. D
2. A
3. A
4. B
5. D
6. A
7. D
8. C
9. D
10. B
11. C
12. D

Section 3

Cognitive Assessment

"The CMT credential has been nothing but good for my career in medical transcription. It has opened doors for me that quite possibly would have been closed without it. Even after I moved from production transcription positions to other facets of the business, having the CMT credential has proven beneficial in a number of ways. As a consultant the CMT provided a level of credibility that offered an extra level of comfort and assurance to prospective clients. In my current position working with the sales team and heading up new client implementations, having the CMT credential has proven extremely helpful in dealing with MT/HIM directors and practice managers." – Jay Vance, CMT

CMT Practice Test

"Use your gifts faithfully, and they shall be enlarged; practice what you know, and you shall attain to higher knowledge."

– Matthew Arnold

Instructions

The CMT exam houses 78 cognitive assessment (multiple-choice) questions and 42 audio items. Below you will find a 78-question practice test designed to parallel the weight and balance of objectives on the CMT exam itself. None of the questions below are taken from the exam, but they represent potential content domains under the blue print to which you have now been oriented by this text. They should give you an overall impression of exam scope and format, though AHDI cautions candidates against the presumption that these items alone may be diagnostic or indicative of exam performance. To assist you with identifying weaknesses under specific objectives, the questions here follow the order of the exam blue print, but keep in mind that items on the CMT exam are *randomized* and will not be identified by objective or competency. (Answer key on page 104.)

1. Which of the following is correctly transcribed?

   A. A gated scan revealed ostial plaque.
   B. A gaited scan revealed ostial plaque.
   C. A gated scan revealed osteal plaque.
   D. A gaited scan revealed osteal plaque.

2. Which sentence is correct?

   A. A drug-eluding stent was used.
   B. A drug-eluting stent was used.

C. A drug-eliding stent was used.
D. A drug-alluding stent was used.

3. Choose the correctly transcribed sentence.

A. A Deaver retractor was placed and the abdominal cavity was explored.
B. A Beaver retractor was placed and the abdominal cavity was explored.
C. A Deaver blade was used to create a corneal incision.
D. A Deaver blade was used to create an abdominal incision.

4. What does the abbreviation PEEP stand for?

A. pulmonary end expiratory pressure
B. positive end-expiratory pressure
C. positive end-expiration pressure
D. positive end-expiratory peak

5. Pick the correct abbreviation that stands for flexion, abduction, external rotation, extension.

A. FAERE
B. FLABERE
C. FABERE
D. FAEX

6. What is the correct abbreviation for chronic fatigue and immune dysfunction syndrome?

A. CFIDS
B. CFAIDS
C. CFIMDS
D. CFIDSY

7. Which BUN value is within the normal range?

A. 12
B. 2
C. 122
D. 200

8. What is the significance of a PTH level of 20 pg/mL?

A. It is mildly elevated.
B. It is decreased.
C. It is normal.
D. It is extremely elevated.

9. What is measured when tidal volume is assessed?

A. maximum amount of air a patient can exhale after taking a deep breath
B. volume of air that remains in the lungs at all times
C. volume of the air that the lungs can hold
D. volume of air that can be moved in and out of the lungs during eupnea

10. The BNP level, used during evaluation of patients for CHF, measures what?

A. a polypeptide secreted by the cardiac ventricles
B. average red blood cell production during a specified time frame
C. the presence or absence of neurofibrillary tangles
D. nitrogen in the blood

11. What proportions does an A/G ratio measure?

A. albumin and globulin in urine
B. albumin and globulin in blood
C. hemoglobin A and glucose in blood
D. hemoglobin A and glucose in urine

12. What condition might be present in a patient with an elevated alkaline phosphatase?

A. microcytic anemia
B. glioblastoma
C. biliary obstruction
D. diabetes mellitus

13. A patient with serum calcium of 12 and a phosphate level of 1.8 would likely have which diagnosis?

A. myocardial infarction
B. primary hyperparathyroidism
C. renal failure
D. HIV

14. What laboratory result suggests the presence of acute viral hepatitis?

A. decreased blood glucose
B. increased urine sodium
C. elevated urine chloride
D. elevated AST

15. What condition is suggested by a homocysteine level of 50 mcmol/L?

A. increased risk of clot formation
B. increased risk for ovarian carcinoma
C. increased risk of prostatic carcinoma
D. increased risk of thyrotoxic crisis

16. Which describes the procedure used in a retrograde pyelography?

A. Contrast is injected into the renal calyces.
B. Contrast injected into the urethra is used to visualize the bladder.
C. Contrast is injected into the ureters from an endoscope placed in the bladder.
D. Contrast injected into the bladder is observed as it passes through the urethra.

17. What diagnostic test is typically performed with the patient in a sitting position?

A. bone densitometry
B. electronystagmography
C. intravenous pyelogram
D. cholangiography

18. What kind of diagnostic test is performed when an opaque dye is injected into the salivary glands?

A. barium swallow
B. lymphangiography
C. sialography
D. dacryocystography

19. What substance is used in performing a barium swallow?

A. barium carbonate
B. barium sulfate
C. barium oxide
D. barium peroxide

20. Which imaging study uses an iodine-based contrast material?

A. virtual colonoscopy
B. brain MRI
C. intravenous pyelogram
D. MRA

21. What condition is suggested by an abnormal Wood lamp examination?

A. fungal infection
B. leukemia
C. tuberculosis
D. anemia

22. Which condition suggested by an elevated erythrocyte sedimentation rate?

A. pernicious anemia
B. diabetes mellitus
C. influenza
D. temporal arteritis

23. On an electromyography report, which phrase is correctly expressed?

A. Sensory latency 0.1 mls
B. Sensory latency 0.1 mS

C. Sensory latency 0.1 msec
D. Sensory latency 0.1 mSec

24. Which sentence correctly expresses a radiation dose level during radiotherapy?

A. Starting dose was 900 cGy.
B. Starting dose was 900 CGY.
C. Starting dose was 900 Cgy.
D. Starting dose was cgray.

25. In the picture at the right, what anatomical feature is indicated by the arrow?

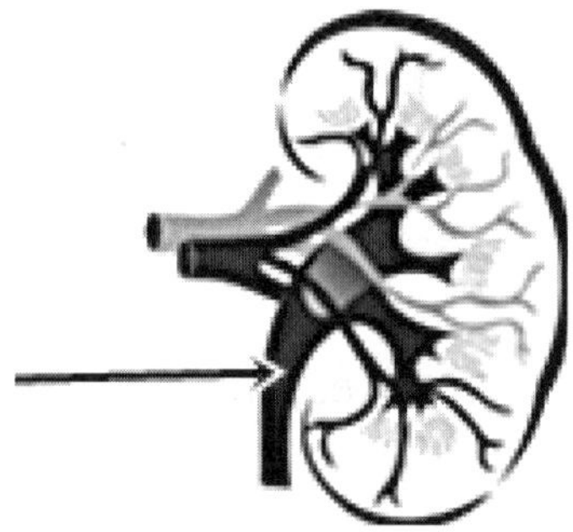

A. common bile duct
B. ureter
C. duodenum
D. renal artery

26. In the picture at the right, what anatomical feature is the arrow pointing to?

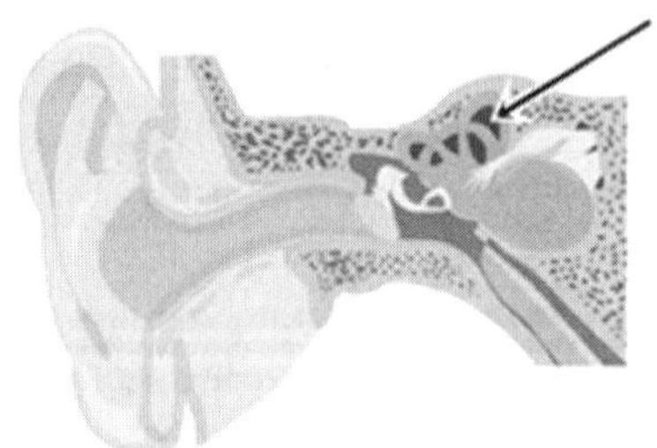

A. incisive canal
B. hypoglossal canals
C. semicircular canals
D. pterygoid canal

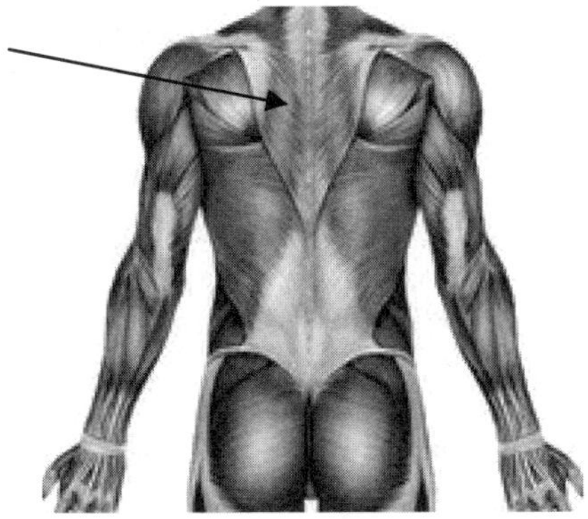

27. What muscle is the arrow above pointing to?

A. deltoid
B. teres major
C. sternocleidomastoid
D. trapezius

28. Which gland is located at the back of the third ventricle of the brain that produces the hormone melatonin?

A. pineal gland
B. pituitary
C. thymus
D. hypothalamus

29. Name the bone that is in the lateral lower arm in line with the thumb.

A. humerus
B. radius
C. ulna
D. tibia

30. Which veins begin near the angle of the mandible and descend through the neck?

A. external jugular
B. vertebral
C. axillary
D. cephalic

31. Which organ is involved in the removal and excretion of metabolic wastes from the blood?

A. liver
B. spleen
C. kidney
D. colon

32. The condition of ascites is the accumulation of fluid where?

A. peritoneal cavity
B. apex of lungs
C. pericardium
D. parietal pleura

33. Which statement about the brain is true?

A. The brain consumes about 80% of the oxygen and glucose used in the body.
B. Large amounts of glucose are stored in the brain.
C. Blood flows to the brain mainly through the internal carotid and vertebral arteries.
D. Proteins and antibiotics easily cross the blood-brain barrier.

34. Abadie sign, or spasm of the levator palpebrae superioris, may be a sign of what condition?

A. hypothyroidism
B. glaucoma
C. hyperthyroidism
D. senile cataract

35. What condition might be indicated by the presence of bruises and petechiae on the extremities?

A. ITP
B. DLE
C. ARDS
D. MAC

36. What condition is suggested by high blood pressure, protein in the urine, and seizures?

A. eclampsia
B. discoid lupus
C. Parkinson disease
D. diabetes insipidus

37. What is a treatment for cystocele?

A. cystectomy
B. colporrhaphy
C. cecostomy
D. chordotomy

38. Pulmonary edema could be treated in what way?

A. tracheotomy and steroid administration
B. nasal cannula oxygen and afterload reduction
C. pneumonectomy and steroid administration
D. pulmonary valve repair and preload reduction

39. Which condition might be treated with an ileal conduit?

A. early-stage colon carcinoma
B. avascular necrosis
C. absence of the urinary bladder after surgery
D. iatrogenic lymphedema

40. For what condition is Benicar prescribed?

A. hypotension
B. type 2 diabetes
C. breast cancer
D. hypertension

41. What class of drugs might be used to treat thrombocytopenia?

A. alpha blocker
B. corticosteroid

C. cephalosporin
D. vasopressor

42. Casodex might be used to treat what disease?

A. prostatitis
B. urinary tract infection
C. metastatic prostate cancer
D. epididymitis

43. **On x-ray, the radiologist reports a widening at the acromioclavicular joint, suggesting the possibility of __________, and followup films are recommended.**

Which condition is likely to be named in the blank?

A. separation
B. carcinoma
C. arthritis
D. crush injury

44. **This 60-year-old woman presents with acute onset of respiratory distress 5 days following colectomy for colon carcinoma. We will order a lung V/Q scan and _____________.**

Which phrase is most likely to fill in the blank?

A. begin chest physiotherapy
B. initiate antibiotic therapy
C. perform immediate bronchoscopy
D. consider starting heparin

45. **This 70-year-old male complains of feeling he cannot empty his bladder completely. He has noted ____ urethral discharge. I have discussed with him that this is likely BPH.**

Which is the most likely word or phrase to fill in the above blank?

A. a greenish
B. no

C. profuse
D. some purulent

46. **This patient presented with symptoms of intermittent crampy abdominal pain, bilious vomiting, and ______. The differential diagnosis includes mechanical bowel obstruction.**

Which phrase would be likely to fill in the above blank?

A. epigastric tenderness
B. marked icterus
C. light-colored stool
D. a history of laparotomy

47. Which are examples of correct classification of cervical intraepithelial neoplasias?

A. CIN1, CIN2
B. CIN-A, CIN-B
C. CIN-I, CIN-II
D. CIN-1, CIN-2

48. In the Binet leukemia classification system, which is the correct expression to describe a case with fewer than 3 areas of enlarged lymphoid tissue?

A. Binet grade 1
B. Binet level 1
C. Binet stage A
D. Binet stage I

49. Which is the correct expression for classifying adenocarcinoma of the prostate?

A. Gleason grade 6
B. Gleason stage VI
C. Gleason score 6
D. Gleason level 6

50. What does a Rancho Los Amigos score of VIII signify?

A. purposeful and appropriate behavior
B. inresponsiveness
C. confused and agitated behavior
D. generalized response to stimuli

51. A patient with a MELD score of 19-24 may be a candidate for what procedure?

A. knee replacement
B. heart transplant
C. cataract surgery
D. liver transplant

52. What kind of surgery would use a columellar chevron incision?

A. angioplasty
B. open rhinoplasty
C. adenoidectomy
D. cataract extraction

53. Seldinger technique would be used in which procedure?

A. heart catheterization
B. lithotripsy
C. stereotactic radiosurgery
D. cesarean section

54. Which procedure places the patient in a flank position and uses an incision overlying the 12th rib?

A. appendectomy
B. colectomy
C. nephrectomy
D. distal pancreatectomy

55. In what kind of surgical procedure might a Bookwalter retractor be used?

A. catheter extraction
B. transsphenoidal resection
C. total hip replacement
D. laparotomy

56. Which type of scissors might be used in vascular surgery?

A. Potts
B. Mayo
C. Stevens
D. bandage

57. Which is a brand of electrocautery device used for hemostasis?

A. DePuy
B. ElecSys
C. Bugbee
D. Arctic

58. In what type of procedure would you find an Angio-Seal used?

A. total hip arthroplasty
B. cardiac catheterization
C. carotid artery stenting
D. rhinoplasty

59. **For placement over the dorsum, a cartilage crusher was used to crush and flatten a small piece of septal cartilage, then the contour was checked and confirmed to be satisfactory.**

Which surgical procedure would contain the above language?

A. rhinoplasty
B. tracheotomy
C. cervical diskectomy
D. myringotomy

60. **The medial borders of the longus colli muscles were dissected free from their attachments. A needle was placed and an x-ray properly localized the space.**

In which surgical procedure would you find the sentences above?

A. anterior cervical diskectomy
B. Achilles tendon repair
C. rhytidectomy
D. thyroidectomy

61. **Needles were passed with direct palpation through the vaginal incision from the lateral thigh to the vaginal incision.**

Which operative report would include the above sentence?

A. hysterectomy
B. cystectomy
C. urethral sling
D. vulvectomy

62. Which abbreviation refers to software used by physicians for direct entry of patient treatment information?

A. CDR
B. PACS
C. OCR
D. CPOE

63. DICOM is the interoperability standard established to support distribution and access to which of these?

A. e-prescriptions
B. imaging studies
C. laboratory data
D. home health reports

64. In the abbreviation ICD-10, what does the "D" refer to?

A. disease
B. diagnosis
C. division
D. diagnostics

65. Which term is used to describe a computer system that is old and outdated?

A. archive
B. legacy
C. sunset
D. next gen

66. Which refers to the application of computer technology to the management of information?

A. integration
B. interoperability
C. informatics
D. implementation

67. Which term describes the kind of health data created from narrative dictation?

A. mineable
B. unstructured
C. discrete
D. abstracted

68. What does the "CT" refer to in SNOMED-CT?

A. computerized tracking
B. clinical technology
C. clinical terms
D. computerized terminology

69. What does the phrase *meaningful use* refer to?

A. Appropriate application of clinical coding standards to avoid fraud and abuse in patient billing.
B. Adoption and integration of EHR systems in a manner that drives coordinated use of health information and improved care outcomes.
C. Capture of core measures information that will generate useable statistical data to support the management of specific diseases.
D. Integration of e-prescribing technologies that eliminate drug-related data entry errors.

70. Which refers to the application of natural language processing using a clinical nomenclature system, such as SNOMED-CT?

A. data tagging
B. data mining
C. data abstracting
D. data integration

71. Which refers to the transcribed document *after* the application of NLP?

A. data file
B. codified narrative
C. abstracted dictation
D. source file

72. The "once-and-done" concept is utilized with which of the following?

A. point-and-click template systems
B. front-end speech recognition
C. back-end speech recognition
D. at the point of authentication of the record

73. Which of the following factors most influences a successful SRT implementation?

A. the type of technology being implemented
B. lack of efficient editing skills
C. inability to resolve style conflicts
D. inconsistency of a dictator's speech pattern

74. An SRT draft document showing exam findings post spontaneous vaginal delivery contains the sentence, "There were no noted peroneal abrasions or lacerations." The MT editor should:

A. Correct "peroneal" to "perineal" and send the report.
B. Leave the report as is and send for physician signature.
C. Flag for physician to clarify.
D. Leave the sentence as is, adding [sic] to indicate verbatim.

75. According to the Book of Style, which elements entered or captured in an electronic environment may not translate correctly?

A. demographic information
B. drug dosages
C. report templates
D. use of certain symbols and styles

76. What does the P in NLP stand for?

A. practitioner
B. processing
C. planning
D. productivity

77. Which of the following would edit front-end SRT?

A. certified medical transcriptionist/editor
B. certified physician's assistant
C. physician
D. QA specialist

78. ROI of technology integration will be successful with results that show:

A. 40% savings in transcription production costs.
B. Amortization of hardware and software costs.
C. Dictators maintaining more than 80% consistency in their speech pattern.
D. Measurable productivity gains.

CMT Practice Test Answer Key

1. A
2. B
3. A
4. B
5. C
6. A
7. A
8. C
9. D
10. A
11. B
12. C
13. B
14. D
15. A
16. C
17. B
18. C
19. B
20. C
21. A
22. D
23. C
24. A
25. B
26. C
27. D
28. A
29. B
30. A
31. C
32. A
33. C
34. C
35. A
36. A

37. B
38. B
39. C
40. D
41. B
42. C
43. A
44. D
45. B
46. D
47. D
48. C
49. C
50. A
51. D
52. B
53. A
54. C
55. D
56. A
57. C
58. B
59. A
60. A
61. C
62. D
63. B
64. A
65. B
66. C
67. B
68. C
69. B
70. A
71. B
72. B
73. D
74. A
75. D
76. B

77. C

78. D

Appendices

Appendix A – CMT Recommended Resources List

The following is a resource list for all the texts cited in this book that are recommended for exam preparation and focused study.

Case Files® Surgery, Third Edition
Author: Eugene Toy, MD; Terrence Liu, MD; Andre Campbell, MD
Publisher: McGraw-Hill Companies, Inc.
©2009
Order: www.mhhe.com

EHR Glossary
Author: Lea Sims, CMT, AHDI-F
Publisher: Association for Healthcare Documentation Integrity
©2011
Order: Included in Appendix D

Ethical Best Practices: Resource Guide for Healthcare Documentation Specialists
Publisher: Association for Healthcare Documentation Integrity
©2010
Order: www.ahdionline.org

Human Diseases, Third Edition
Author: John H. Dirckx, MD
Publisher: Health Professions Institute
©2009
Order: www.hpisum.com

Laboratory Tests and Diagnostic Procedures in Medicine
Author: John H. Dirckx, MD
Publisher: Health Professions Institute
©2004
Order: www.hpisum.com

Medline Plus Videos of Surgical Procedures
Provider: U.S. National Library of Medicine/National Institutes of Health
View: http://www.nlm.nih.gov/medlineplus/surgeryvideos.html

Principles of Human Anatomy, 12th Edition
Author: Gerard. J. Tortora and Mark T. Nielsen
Publisher: John Wiley and Sons, Inc.
©2011
Order: www.wiley.com

Quick Look Drug Book 2011
Author: Leonard L. Lance, RPh, BSPharm
Publisher: Wolters Kluwer Health / Lippincott Williams & Wilkins
©2011
Order: www.stedmans.com

Speech Recognition Editing Course Online
Contributors: Association for Healthcare Documentation Integrity; TRS Institute; 3M Health Information Services
Order: www.ahdionline.org

Stedman's Medical Dictionary for the Health Professions and Nursing, 6th Edition, Illustrated
Publisher: Wolters Kluwer Health / Lippincott Williams & Wilkins
©2011
Order: www.stedmans.com

Technology for the Medical Transcriptionist
Author: Laura Bryan, MT, (ASCP), CMT, AHDI-F
Publisher: Wolters Kluwer Health / Lippincott Williams & Wilkins
©2010
Order: www.stedmans.com

The Book of Style for Medical Transcription, Third Edition
Author: Lea Sims, CMT, AHDI-F
Publisher: Association for Healthcare Documentation Integrity
©2008
Order: www.ahdionline.org

The CMT Review Guide
Author: Betty Honkonen, CMT, AHDI-F
Publisher: Wolters Kluwer Health / Lippincott Williams & Wilkins
©2005
www.stedmans.com

The Language of Medicine, 9th Edition
Author: Davi-Ellen Chabner, BA, MAT
Publisher: Elsevier, Inc.
©2011
Order: www.us.elsevierhealth.com

Using Medical Terminology: A Practical Approach
Author: Judi.L. Nath, PhD
©2005
Publisher: Wolters Kluwer Health / Lippincott Williams & Wilkins
Order: www.stedmans.com

Appendix B - Credentialing Overview

AHDI offers two voluntary credentials for medical transcription practitioners:

- Registered Medical Transcriptionist (RMT) – Level 1
- Certified Medical Transcriptionist (CMT) – Level 2

AHDI offers voluntary credentialing exams to individuals who wish to demonstrate job readiness and level-specific competency to prospective employers, clients, and industry colleagues. In offering credentialing exams for medical transcriptionists, AHDI is protecting the public interest by promoting professional standards, improving the practice of medical transcription, and recognizing those professionals who demonstrate competency through the fulfillment of stated requirements.

AHDI exams are delivered by Kryterion, a full-service test development and delivery company that provides world-class online testing technology integrating item banking, test delivery, and real-time reports; while leveraging a global network of testing centers. Kryterion is the market leader in live Online Proctoring (OLP), which utilizes remote video monitoring to observe test takers where they live, learn, or work.

The credentialing department at AHDI determines individual eligibility for exam admission. Based on test specifications developed by AHDI, Kryterion prepares and administers the individual tests approved by AHDI. Kryterion is also responsible for procuring and maintaining testing sites and overseeing online proctoring, test security, test administration, and related functions.

Visit the AHDI website at www.ahdionline.org and click on "Certification" for complete exam information and pricing. Interested persons should download and review the complete Credentialing Candidate Guide before scheduling your exam.

Appendix C - CMT Exam Blue Print Checklist

CMT candidates preparing for access to the CMT exam should adopt a study approach that incorporates preparation against the exam blue print. All questions a candidate will encounter on the CMT exam were strictly written against this blue print. Use the following checklist to assist you as you study each competency domain, marking the check box for each objective when you feel you have mastered the objective and have a strong working knowledge of concepts and information tha t fall within that domain area.

Section 1	Clinical Medicine	Studied Content Resources?	Completed Assessments?
1.1	Given a sentence, identify the correct use of a commonly confused medical term.		
1.2	Given an audio excerpt containing a clinical term, correctly transcribe the excerpt, <u>or</u> given an excerpt with transcribed text, fill in the blank(s) representing omitted information.		
1.3	Given a laboratory result, identify if the value is low, high, or normal.		
1.4	Given an audio excerpt containing a laboratory term, correctly transcribe the excerpt, <u>or</u> given an excerpt with transcribed text, fill in the blank(s) representing omitted information.		
1.5	Given an imaging study, identify processes, technologies, and patient positions used in that study.		
1.6	Given an imaging study, identify common contrast media used in that study.		
1.7	Given imaging study results or values, identify the associated disease or diagnosis, <u>or</u> given a disease or diagnosis, identify the associated imaging study results or values.		

1.8	Given unique imaging study values, identify the correct expression or definition of the values.		
1.9	Given an audio excerpt containing an imaging term, correctly transcribe the excerpt, or given an excerpt with transcribed text, fill in the blank(s) representing omitted information.		
1.10	Given an audio excerpt containing a pharmacology term, correctly transcribe the excerpt, or given an excerpt with transcribed text, fill in the blank(s) representing omitted information.		
1.11	Given an abbreviation, identify the correct term, or given a term, identify the correct abbreviation.		
1.12	Given an audio excerpt containing any clinical term or abbreviation from a medical specialty, fill in the blank(s) representing omitted information.		
1.13	Given a graphic showing anatomy or systems, identify the anatomy or system.		
1.14	Given a position or location, identify the anatomical part of the human body.		
1.15	Given a physiologic process, identify the steps or functions related to that process.		
1.16	Given a sign or symptom, identify the disease or syndrome, or given a disease or syndrome, identify the sign or symptom.		
1.17	Given a disease or syndrome, identify the treatment course.		
1.18	Given a diagnostic test including laboratory studies, identify what is being measured.		
1.19	Given laboratory test results or values, identify the associated disease or diagnosis, or given a disease or diagnosis, identify		

	the associated laboratory test results or values.		
1.20	Given an audio excerpt containing a diagnostic test, fill in the blank(s) representing omitted information.		
1.21	Given a medication, identify the symptom or disease for which it is prescribed, <u>or</u> given a symptom or disease, identify the medication that is prescribed.		
1.22	Given a diagnostic scenario that could include signs/symptoms, physical exam findings, diagnostic test results, and diagnosis, identify information about the signs/symptoms, physical exam findings, diagnostics test results, and diagnosis.		
1.23	Given a classification system, identify the expressed score or grade.		
1.24	Given a classification system result, identify the disease or affected anatomical part.		
1.25	Given a surgical approach or technique (anesthesia, positions, incisions, suture techniques, etc), identify the procedure with which it is associated.		
1.26	Given surgical equipment or a surgical instrument, identify the procedure with which it is associated.		
1.27	Given an excerpt from an operative report, identify the procedure that was conducted.		
1.28	Given an audio excerpt containing a classification system or treatment term, fill in the blank(s) representing omitted information.		

Section 2	Health Information Technology	Studied Content Resources?	Completed Assessments?
2.1	Given an abbreviation, identify the correctly expanded form.		
2.2	Given an EHR technology term, identify the correct definition, or given a definition, identify the correct EHR technology term.		
2.3	Given an SRT term or concept, identify the correct definition, or given a definition, identify the correct SRT term or concept.		
2.4	Given a list, identify success factors for SRT adoption/integration as defined by the Book of Style.		
2.5	Given scenarios, identify the correct application of Book of Style standards for resolving style conflicts in an SRT editing environment.		
2.7	Given a term or concept related to nomenclatures or measurement systems, identify the correct definition.		
2.8	Given a term or concept related to NLP, identify the correct definition.		

Appendix D – EHR Glossary

Below you will find a glossary of terms related to electronic medical records, electronic health records, and health information technology.

Addendum	Text that is added to a document after it has been finalized.
Alerts	Pop-ups or reminders. An automated warning system such a clinical alerts, preventive health maintenance, medication interactions etc.
Ambulatory Care	Medical care provided on an outpatient basis.
Annotator	A system function that allows an explanatory note or diagram to be added to an image.
ASP **Application Service Provider**	An Application Service Provider (ASP) is a third-party entity that deploys, hosts and manages software from a centrally managed host facility (offsite). Applications are delivered over networks (WAN, Internet) on a subscription fee/rental basis. This model is also been referred to as "software-as-a-service."
Audit Trail	Security system that tracks a user's access, deletion, or modification of data. The term used in healthcare information security refers to a chronological record of system resource usage. This includes user login, file access, other various activities, and whether any actual or attempted security violations occurred, legitimate or unauthorized.
Authentication	The verification of the identity of a person or process.
Bandwidth	A data transmission rate; the maximum amount of

	information (bits/second) that can be transmitted along a channel.
Bar Code	A printed horizontal strip of vertical bars which represent decimal digits used for identification. Bar codes must be read by a bar code reader.
Biometrics	Biometrics are automated methods of recognizing a person based on a physiological characteristic such as fingerprints, retina, voice etc.
Browser	Short for Web browser, a software application used to locate and display Web pages.
Case Management	A process of identifying individuals at high risk for problems associated with complex health care needs and assessing opportunities to coordinate care to optimize the outcome.
Chart	Medical record
Chart Note	A document, written by the clinician or provider, which describes the details of a patient's encounter. Sometimes referred to as a progress note.
Client/Server architecture	An information-transmission arrangement, in which a client program sends a request to a server. When the server receives the request, it disconnects from the client and processes the request. When the request is processed, the server reconnects to the client program and the information is transferred to the client. This usually implies that the server is located on site as opposed to the ASP (Application Server Provider) architecture.
Clinical Data Repository (CDR)	A real-time database that consolidates data from a variety of clinical sources to present a unified view of a single

	patient. It is optimized to allow clinicians to retrieve data for a single patient rather than to identify a population of patients with common characteristics or to facilitate the management of a specific clinical department.
Clinical Decision support system (CDSS)	A clinical decision support system (CDSS) is software designed to aid clinicians in decision making by matching individual patient characteristics to computerized knowledge bases for the purpose of generating patient-specific assessments or recommendations.
Clinical Guidelines (Protocols)	Clinical guidelines are recommendations based on the latest available evidence for the appropriate treatment and care of a patient's condition.
Clinical messaging	Communication of clinical information within the electronic medical record to other healthcare personnel.
CPG	Clinical Practice Guidelines
CPM	Clinical Performance Measures
CPOE Computerized Provider Order Entry	CPOE refers to the act of a clinician entering an order for patient services into an information system.
CPR Computerized Patient Record, Computer-Based Patient Record	Electronically maintained information about an individual's lifetime health status and healthcare from all specialties.
CPT Current Procedural Terminology	The purpose of CPT codes is to provide a uniform language that accurately describes medical, surgical, and diagnostic services.
Data conversion	The conversion of data from one software to another.

Data Encryption Standard (DES)	Data Encryption Standard (DES) is a widely-used method of data encryption using a private (secret) key.
Data Integrity	Refers to the validity of data. A condition in which data has not been altered or destroyed in an unauthorized manner.
Data Mining	The process of analyzing or extracting data from a database to identify patterns or relationships.
Data Set	A group of data elements relevant for a particular use.
Data Structure	A way to store and organize data in order to facilitate access and modifications.
Database	A collection of information organized in such a way that a computer program can quickly select desired pieces of data.
Database management system (DBMS)	A set of computer programs for organizing the information in a database. A DBMS supports the structuring of the database in a standard format and provides tools for data input, verification, storage, retrieval, query, and manipulation.
DICOM Digital Imaging and Communications in Medicine	Digital Imaging and Communications in Medicine (DICOM) is a standard to aid the distribution and viewing of medical images, such as CT scans, MRIs, and ultrasound.
Dictation	The process by which a physician records his/her notes about a patient. This recording is intended for reproduction in written word (transcription).
Digital Signature	Sometimes referred to as Advanced Electronic Signature. Digital signature takes the traditional hand-written signature and creates a digital image of the signature to

	eliminate the need to print and sign documents.
Discrete Data	A set of data is said to be discrete if the values belonging to it are distinct and separate, (i.e., they can be counted). Discrete data is more easily reportable as opposed to non-discrete or unstructured data.
Document Imaging	Converting paper documents into an electronic format usually through a scanning process.
Documentation	The process of recording information.
Document Management	Is a system involving scanning, categorizing and storing vital patient documents.
DOQ-IT Doctors Office Quality Information Technology	DOQ-IT is a two-year special study that is designed to improve quality of care, patient safety, and efficiency for services provided to Medicare beneficiaries by promoting the adoption of EHR's and Information Technology (IT) in primary care physician offices.
E & M Coding Evaluation and Management Coding	Documentation guidelines for Evaluation and Management CPT codes from the Center for Medicare and Medicaid Services (formerly HCFA).
EDI	Electronic Data Interchange
EHR Electronic Health Record	An electronic repository of information regarding the health of an individual. It is also a generic term for all electronic patient care systems. E HR's imply a level of interoperability beyond the capability of an EMR (Electronic Medical Record).
Electronic Superbill	An electronic encounter form used for coding and billing.

EMR Electronic Medical Record	Electronic Medical record has a level of sophistication beyond a document management system. An EMR is a provider-based medical record that includes all health documentation for one person covering all services provided within an enterprise.
EOE Electronic Order Entry	The function of this program is to move from hand-written and verbal orders to computer-based entry.
EPR Electronic Patient Record	Same as a CPR – Computerized Patient Record.
Encryption	Process of converting messages or data into a form that cannot be read without decrypting or deciphering it.
e-Prescribing	Prescribing medication through an automated data-entry process and transmitting the information to participating pharmacies.
Evidence based medicine	Evidence-based medicine (EBM) is the integration of best research evidence with clinical expertise to aid in the diagnosis and management of patients.
Face Sheet	Also called a Summary Screen or Patient Dashboard. This screen includes a summary of patient relevant information on one screen.
Fat Client	A fat client is a network computer with a hard disc drive, as opposed to a thin client which has no disc drive.
Firewall	A system designed to prevent unauthorized access to or from a private computer network.
Formulary	A listing of prescription drugs established by a particular health plan which includes both Brand name and Generic

	drugs. It serves to suggest covered, preferred and lower cost drugs.
FTP	File Transfer Program
Graphical User Interface (GUI)	Abbreviated GUI .A program interface that takes advantage of the computer's graphics capabilities to make the program easier to use. Well-designed graphical user interfaces can help expedite the software learning process.
Help Desk	Service and support desk
HIPAA Health Insurance Portability and Accountability Act	HIPAA seeks to establish standardized mechanisms for electronic data interchange (EDI), security, and confidentiality of all healthcare-related data.
HL7 Health Level 7	Formed in the United States in 1987, HL7 has the goal of developing an international set of open standards for data format and content that allows different health information systems to easily and effectively communicate with one another.
Hot Keys	One- or two-keystroke command that switches the user to a different program or function within a software program. Hot keys are useful to expedite movement within a software program.
HM Health Maintenance	Health Maintenance, also referred to as Preventive Health Maintenance is a system of guidelines (recommended schedules) of tests or procedures that have proven value in disease prevention.
ICD-9 or ICD-10 International Classification of Diseases	ICD is the classification and coding of diseases and injuries.

Informatics	The application of computer technology to the management of information.
Integration	Integration allows for secure communication between enterprise applications.
Interoperability	The capability to provide successful communication between end-users across a mixed environment of different domains, networks, facilities and equipment.
ISP	Internet Service Provider
IT Information Technology	The development, installation, and implementation of computer systems and applications.
Kiosk	Small computer workstations which allow information to be input. Patient kiosks are used for patients to input information into the system at the medical practice, usually input through a workstation in the waiting room.
LAN Local Area Network	A LAN supplies networking capability to a group of computers in close proximity to each other such as in an office building, a school, or a home.
Legacy System	A system that is considered old and possibly out-dated.
Legacy System Integration	The integration of data between a legacy system and some other software program most commonly using HL-7 standards.
LEPR Longitudinal Patient Record	Longitudinal Patient Record is an EHR that includes all healthcare information from all sources.
Macro	A symbol, name or key (macro key) that represents a list of commands, actions, keystrokes or blocks of text. When the

	macro key code is typed, the program carries out the instructions of the macro. Users create macros to save time by replacing often-used, series of strokes (blocks of text) with quick macro key codes.
Network	A system for communication among two or more computers.
OCR Optical Character Recognition	OCR is recognition of printed or written characters by a computer.
PACS Picture Archiving and Communication System	An information system for the storage and distribution of digital radiology images over a networked environment that allows for instant access to images and reports.
Patient Portal	Allow patients and providers to communicate over the Internet in a secure environment.
PDA Personal Desk Assistant or Personal Digital Assistant.	PDA is a hand-held device with a multitude of uses such as scheduling appointments on a calendar, creating to-do lists, storing libraries of medical information, viewing patient specific data . PDA allow for mobility. They are also referred to as palmtops, hand-held computers and pocket computers.
PHI	Protected Health Information
PHM	Preventive Health Maintenance – see Health Maintenance.
PHR – Personal Health Record	A PHR includes all healthcare information from all sources, compiled and maintained by the patient.
Platform	The basic technology of a computer system's hardware and software that defines how a computer is operated and determines what other kinds of software can be used.

PM	Practice Management (billing) system.
PMRI	Patient Medical Record Information
PMS	Practice Management System
Point and Click	Allowing the activation of commands by moving the cursor over certain areas or icons and clicking a pointing device.
Point-of-Care	POC refers to the time while with the patient, either bedside or during an encounter.
Portal	A website considered as an entry point to other websites. Examples are a Patient Portal.
Problem List	Diagnosis list
Protocols	Clinical Guidelines
Pull Down Menu	Also called a drop-down menu. These are a menu of commands or options that appears when you select an item with a mouse.
QIO Quality Improvement Organization	The Medicare QIO program consists of a national network of fifty-three QIO's found in each state responsible to work with consumers, physicians, hospitals, and other caregivers to refine care delivery systems. They are associated with the DOQ-IT program.
Query	The primary mechanism for retrieving information from a database and consists of questions presented to the database in a predefined format.
RFID	Radio Frequency Identification

ROI – Return on Investment	Return on investment typically means measuring an increase in revenue, a decrease in expense or an avoidance of expense.
Scalable	Refers to how well a hardware or software system can adapt to increased demands.
Security	Is the effort to create a secure computing platform, designed so that agents (users or programs) can only perform actions that have been allowed.
Server Farm	A group of networked servers that are housed in one location.
Single sign-on	(SSO) is mechanism whereby a single action of user authentication and authorization can permit a user to access all computers and systems where he/she has access permission, without the need to enter multiple passwords.
SNOMED CT® Systematized Nomenclature of Medicine – Clinical Terms	SNOMED CT ® is a clinical, health care terminology and infrastructure. SNOMED CT ® contains over 366,170 health care concepts with unique meanings and formal logic-based definitions organized into hierarchies.
SOAP note format	A format for medical documentation. SOAP is an acronym for S-Subjective, O-Objective, A-Assessment, P-Plan.
Speech Recognition	The ability of a computer to understand the spoken word for the purpose of receiving commands and transforming speech into text.
Structured Data	Structured data is managed by technology that allows for querying and reporting against predetermined data types and understood relationships.

T1 Line	The T1 carrier is a commonly used digital Internet connection line in the US supporting data rates of 1.544Mbits per second.
Tablet PC	A tablet PC is a computer shaped in the form of a notebook except it has the capabilities of being written on through the use of digitizing tablet technology or a touch screen. A user can use a stylus and operate the computer without having to have a keyboard or mouse.
Template	Often called a library or dictionary. Templates are pre-defined choices of pick-lists designed to streamline the documentation process.
Thin Client	A thin client is a network computer without a hard disc drive, as opposed to a fat client which includes a disc drive.
Transcription	The process by which medical transcriptionists convert physician's dictation into written (typed) words.
Touch Screen	An input device that allows user to interact with the computer by touching the display screen.
Unstructured Data	Data which is not structured such as free-text. The computer cannot automatically extract properties and relationships from unstructured data.
Voice Recognition	See Speech Recognition
VPN - Virtual Private Network	A way to communicate through a dedicated server securely to a corporate network over the internet.
WAN Wide Area Network	A computer network that spans a larger geographical area than a LAN (Local Area Network).

Webinar	A lecture, presentation, workshop or seminar that is transmitted over the Web. Short for Web-based Seminar.
Web Portal	A website considered as an entry point to other websites.
Wireless	A system employing no connecting wire between the transmitting and receiving stations.
Workflow	The automation of a process, in whole or part, during which documents, information or tasks are passed from one participant to another for action, according to a set of procedural rules.

Appendix E – AHDI Membership

The Association for Healthcare Documentation Integrity (AHDI) is a not-for-profit professional association incorporated in California in February 1978, with headquarters in Modesto, California. AHDI offers information about the profession of medical transcription, provides continuing education for medical transcriptionists, and enhances communication among those allied with the profession of medical transcription.

There are a number of resources available to the healthcare documentation expert in today's Internet age. More than ever before, an MT has access to new terminology, advances in clinical medicine, and changes and trends in the industry through online networking. But these resources cannot fully inform or prepare the conscientious practitioner for trends, drivers, and changes in any industry. Navigating the sea of information related to technology, standards, professional development, etc., can be difficult to manage alone. Associations exist to provide practitioners of a given industry the opportunity to work in concert toward the same goals.

AHDI offers its practitioners the opportunity for and access to resources, information, events, and services that empower them to make informed choices that lead to successful career outcomes. Together, we work to advance the profession through legislative advocacy, standard-setting, and professional development.

While AHDI members receive many tangible benefits (publications, discounts, etc.), the decision to become a member of any professional association should be based on more than a desire for tangible benefits. The decision to commit your personal resources toward AHDI membership should reflect the following:

- Support of the mission, goals and objectives of the organization
- Desire to become part of a proactive body of practitioners working toward advancing the profession and driving change in the industry
- Need for information, services, products, and programs that will empower you as a practitioner
- Need for networking and personnel connection with your industry peers, particularly if you are an at-home, isolated practitioner

Find out more about AHDI and sign up online today by visiting our website – www.ahdionline.org or calling our toll free number 800-982-2182.

Appendix F – AHDI Product Highlights

The Book of Style for Medical Transcription, 3rd edition

$50.00 members
$70.00 nonmembers

The 3rd edition of The Book of Style for Medical Transcription from the Association for Healthcare Documentation Integrity (AHDI) is now available in print and in a web-based electronic version. This widely acclaimed industry standards manual has long been the trusted resource for data capture and documentation standards in healthcare. The 3rd edition delivers a streamlined and strategically reorganized flow of critical data, enhanced explanation of standards and practical application, robust examples taken from clinical medicine settings, and so much more.

The Book of Style Workbook

$35.00 members
$50.00 nonmembers

This companion workbook to The Book of Style for Medical Transcription, 3rd edition, is designed to work in tandem with the Book of Style.
The Workbook contains practical application exercises to assist students, postgraduates, and working MTs with orientation to standards and preparation for AHDI credentialing exams.

Mega MT Challenge I & II

$35.00 members, $45.00 nonmembers (Each individual CD)
$60.00 members, $80.00 nonmembers **(Combo Deal)**

These electronic CDs contain over 1200 questions (combined) related to the practice of medical transcription. You'll find questions pertaining to medical terminology, English fundamentals, pharmacology, and an array of medical specialties. A broad variety of question formats (including multiple-choice, true/false, circle one, fill in the blank, etc.) are designed to fully test the wealth of knowledge essential to the practice of transcription. Whether used for self-study, exam preparation, evaluation, staff training, potential employee testing, or classroom instruction, these products are designed to help meet those needs. Order online or by phone.

CMT Prep Quizzes, Volume I, II, III

$25.00 members (each CD)
$35.00 nonmembers (each CD)
Bundle Pricing Available Online

Each CD contains a whopping 240 exam-style questions, answers, and descriptions as found in archived publications. This interactive CD allows you to take the quiz on screen, view the answers and descriptions Makes for great level II prep questions, as well as practice with on-screen test taking. Order online or by phone.

Willie Getwell

$25.00 members
$35.00 nonmembers

This CD provides proofreading and editing exercises designed to enhance your skill in the area of editing and error recognition. You will find 40 transcribed and speech-recognized drafts to orient you to the unique editing and proofing process associated with both domains. Product is perfect for getting your editing up to speed before testing. Order online or by phone.

CMT Prep Assessment Online Course

$100.00 members
$125.00 nonmembers

Offered every month of the year, this four-week course is designed to assist individuals preparing for the CMT exam. Course offers assessment in over 20 body systems. Each body system covered will list websites, medical texts, and references from *The Book of Style for Medical Transcription, 3e,* where applicable. Register online or by phone.

Ethical Best Practices: Resource Guide for Healthcare Documentation Specialists

$70 members
$100 nonmembers

The guide contains all content from the original *Ethical Best Practices Manual for the Healthcare Documentation Sector* that relates specifically to best practices for our workforce. Practice guidelines related to at-home HIPAA and regulatory compliance, compensation, employee vs. independent contractor status, and provision of services are all included in this resource guide for the working MT. Sample agreements and contracts, including business associate and noncompete/nonsolicitation agreements are included.

Note: This is a smaller supplement designed for medical transcriptionists and does not contain all contracts, guidelines, and customizable forms contained in the full Manual. MTSOs and independent contractors should refer to the full EBP Manual.

Medicolegal Flashcards

$25.00 members
$35.00 nonmembers

AHDI ***Flash Cards*** are designed to provide the student, new graduate, and/or seasoned MT with quick, high-impact study tools for skill-building and exam preparation. Take this handy, convenient pack of easy-to-use flash cards with you when you travel, have a long wait in a doctor's office or kids' soccer practice, or just need to make the most of that 10 minutes between appointments. Each set of flashcards covers a content area on the AHDI exam blueprint and is designed to put that core knowledge right at your fingertips. This set of medicolegal flash cards will test your knowledge and understanding of a broad range of medicolegal concepts and terms associated with the healthcare delivery and the documentation sector including such topics as: ***HIPAA, document types, document formats, the legal record, malpractice, DNRs***, and many more.

TO ORDER ANY PRODUCT ABOVE, VISIT WWW.AHDIONLINE.ORG. You can also call AHDI at 1-800-982-2182 to place an order by phone.